"This is a terrific book! In twelve detailed, vividly authentic case studies, Jakes captures the interactive realities that psychotherapists encounter with clients suffering from psychosis. The reader is invited to observe a master clinician at work, to learn from his example, to listen to what patients say and what he hears in sessions, and to see what he says and does and why. This book is filled with valuable clinical wisdom and practical guidance."

—**Michael Garrett**, *MD, emeritus professor of clinical psychiatry, SUNY Downstate Medical Center, New York; faculty, Psychoanalytic Association of New York*

"The clarity of the writing and the relevance of the case studies allow this way of working with the client with psychosis to be accessible to all mental health professionals. . . . I recommend this book to all clinicians working with clients with medication-resistant psychosis."

—**Doug Turkington,** *MD, FRCPsych, Professor of Psychosocial Psychiatry, NewCastle University; Medical director, Insight CBT partnership*

"Simon Jakes shares his experience of providing therapy for clients report-ing problems described as psychotic. He draws upon both cognitive (CBT) and psychoanalytic ideas and techniques, illustrating how he does so with a wide range of clients. This type of sharing is rare in the field of psy-chotherapy and is particularly rewarding when much of what is written is over-technical, concealing the reality and human dimension of therapy. The theoretical background is first presented in an engaging, informal, and read-ily understandable way. The bulk of the book is taken up with descriptions of individuals he has worked with, intermingling vignettes, therapy dialogue, and discussion of conceptual points, illuminating obstacles in the ongoing relationship. The book will be especially invaluable to novice therapists and will help to counter a biological and reductive view of psychosis."

—**Richard Hallam**, *clinical psychologist, psychotherapist, and independent researcher*

"Drawing on decades of experience in this field, Simon Jakes has written a thought provoking and interesting book that assimilates two distinct styles of therapy in a cogent and innovative way. Combining psychodynamic and cognitive therapies, Jakes uses case studies to illustrate examples of this novel approach to working. This is a highly readable and interesting book and I would recommend it for any therapist who works with this population."

—**Dallas Rae**, *clinical psychologist and former director of allied health and mental health services at Liverpool Hospital*

Using Psychodynamic Thinking to Enhance CBT in Clients with Psychosis

Using Psychodynamic Thinking to Enhance CBT in Clients with Psychosis presents a comprehensive method for linking clients' symptoms to their personal development and life problems.

Using concrete examples and extensive case descriptions that often span many years, the chapters show clinicians how to construct a psychodynamic case conceptualisation and how to then guide the direction of the therapy.

The book will be of interest to experienced clinicians, therapists in training, and anyone looking for an integrative approach to the psychotherapy of clients with psychotic presentations.

Simon Jakes trained in clinical psychology at the Institute of Psychiatry in London, graduating with the M.Phil. degree in 1982. He has provided and supervised CBT for psychosis since the 1990s.

Using Psychodynamic Thinking to Enhance CBT in Clients with Psychosis

A Case Study Guide

Simon Jakes

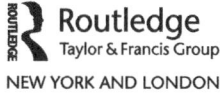
Routledge
Taylor & Francis Group

NEW YORK AND LONDON

Designed cover image: © Getty

First published 2023
by Routledge
605 Third Avenue, New York, NY 10158

and by Routledge
4 Park Square, Milton Park, Abingdon, Oxon, OX14 4RN

Routledge is an imprint of the Taylor & Francis Group, an informa business

© 2023 Simon Jakes

Library of Congress Cataloging-in-Publication Data
Names: Jakes, Simon, 1956- author.
Title: Using psychodynamic thinking to enhance CBT in clients with
    psychosis : a case study guide / Simon Jakes.
Description: New York, NY : Routledge, 2023. | Includes
    bibliographical references and index.
Identifiers: LCCN 2022046668 (print) | LCCN 2022046669
    (ebook) | ISBN 9780367764333 (hardback) | ISBN 9780367764319
    (paperback) | ISBN 9781003168379 (ebook)
Subjects: LCSH: Cognitive therapy. | Psychodynamic psychotherapy. |
    Psychoses—Treatment.
Classification: LCC RC489.C89 J354 2023 (print) | LCC RC489.C89
    (ebook) | DDC 616.89/1425—dc23/eng/20221122
LC record available at https://lccn.loc.gov/2022046668
LC ebook record available at https://lccn.loc.gov/2022046669

ISBN: 978-0-367-76433-3 (hbk)
ISBN: 978-0-367-76431-9 (pbk)
ISBN: 978-1-003-16837-9 (ebk)

DOI: 10.4324/9781003168379

Typeset in Bembo
by Apex CoVantage, LLC

To my parents

Contents

Foreword

This eminently readable and clinically astute book builds on the work of Michael Garrett of the State University of New York who in 2011 described CBT for psychosis as delivered in a psychoanalytic frame. The clarity of the writing and the relevance of the case studies allow this way of working with the client with psychosis to be accessible to all mental health professionals. I am reminded of a quote from Aaron T. Beck, who said, "the clinician is a therapist first and a cognitive therapist second". The author invites us to consider other models of psychosis with a view to enriching our therapeutic skills. One such model struck me from the text. . . . Jung described the unity of the personality as "an illusion" and postulated that we are all made up of "innumerable sub-personalities each with a will of their own". This psychodynamic model made me reconsider the contents of the hundreds of voice diaries I had read over the years and the different voices which were making their point of view heard. Perhaps instead of trying to change the relationship with the entire voice-hearing experience, I could have guided the client to focus on the most meaningful voice. Classical CBT for psychosis is often effective in early intervention settings, but in chronic psychosis, more sessions and a slower pace are clearly needed. The author invites us to take more time building the therapeutic relationship with clients with chronic psychosis/schizophrenia and to gently explore the underlying meaning in the symptoms. He accentuates the importance of pace and of being aware of the counter-transference. I recommend this book to all clinicians working with clients with medication-resistant psychosis.

Dr Doug Turkington, MD, FRCPsych,
Professor of Psychosocial Psychiatry, NewCastle University;
Medical director, Insight CBT partnership

Acknowledgements

I would like to thank Jacky Knibbs, Douglas Turkington, John Rhodes, Richard Hallam, Shirley Chen, Lynda Nguyen, Dallas Rae, Joseph Jakes, Samuel Jakes, and Soraya Issa for their feedback on earlier versions of this text. I would also like to thank Daniela Vladislavic for her unending support in my role as a cognitive therapist in the Youth Team, and Soraya for giving me the space to write the book. I would particularly like to thank all the clients who agreed to have their stories included in the book and also all the people who contributed to these ideas through discussions over the years. These include, but are not limited to, Richard Hallam, John Rhodes, Paul Chadwick, Dallas Rae, Shirley Chen, and Ian Jakes, and, of course, my parents for all their support. Needless to say, none of these people are responsible for any of the mistakes in the text.

1 Introduction

Macbeth's Dagger

This book developed from working with psychotic clients using psychological therapy over the long term. When I first began to use cognitive therapy with psychotic clients, one of the consultant psychiatrists told me that the clients wouldn't come. It turned out that, although this was true for some clients, it wasn't true for others. For some clients, it wasn't that they didn't come, but that they didn't want to stop coming that was the problem. And what could you do for the client after working on their delusional beliefs and coping skills? A minimum of 12 sessions of Cognitive Therapy for Psychosis (CBTp) should be offered to people with Schizophrenia, according to the recommendations in the NICE guidelines for Schizophrenia, but obviously a client with chronic psychosis is unlikely to fully recover in this time. So, should the therapist just stop? Hazel Nelson (1997, 2005) offers clients around a year of therapy, mainly focused on modification of delusions. But what then? And what should we do if the client remains uninterested in questioning whether their delusions are true or false?

In this book, I look at one possible answer to these questions. One can offer a cognitive therapy of a broader type, influenced by psychodynamic ideas. Psychoanalysts these days maintain that the transference is present from the very beginning of the therapy; on the other hand, a client who has been attending for six months clearly has a different relationship to the therapist to one who began attending only last week, and if we see clients for a longer period of time, it is likely that issues around the relationship to the therapist—transference—will develop and will need to be managed. Furthermore, information processing models of working cognitively with psychotic symptoms can portray the clients' problems in a simplified way. One characteristic of CBTp has been the focus on symptoms and scepticism about syndromes. For example, a client hears voices and then interprets these as evidence that he or she is being spied on, and the problem is the negative interpretation that the client makes about the voices. While this can be true, and a worthwhile problem to work on, it is also true that most people who become psychotic have more pervasive difficulties which often make it difficult to engage in life, so it is usually a partial explanation. It is all very well to work on single symptoms, but it is not an accident that many

DOI:10.4324/9781003168379-1

people with delusions or voices have major problems in relating to other people or in working. Thinking about the person psychodynamically is one way of broadening the conceptualisation of the client.

This approach has recently been suggested by Garrett (2019) and Garrett and Turkington (2011). They have suggested that a psychodynamic frame can help to understand psychotic clients in CBT and that additionally, after an initial period of CBT, it is helpful to include a second, psychodynamic, phase of therapy. They present a case study of a client with chronic psychosis whose social functioning improved during the course of therapy over many years. This approach seems hopeful, because it broadens the therapy and can also help to support the therapist in what can be a personally challenging endeavour. This is a welcome approach, because too often different psychotherapies have becoming self-perpetuating closed systems. Therapists in one school often avoid the ideas and methods of therapists in other schools, and psychotherapy loses out from the possibility of cross-fertilisation.

This book is divided into two parts. The first part outlines (1) the main ideas and techniques of cognitive therapy as applied to psychosis (CBTp), (2) the psychodynamic model of psychosis (and alterations to the method that psychoanalysts have made in order to work with psychotic clients) and (3) how some of these psychodynamic ideas and methods might be applied to enrich cognitive therapy. The second part describes in detail the psychotherapy of a number of different clients using CBTp as a base and incorporating psychodynamic ideas and methods. The first part is really to orient therapists not familiar with either cognitive psychotherapy or psychodynamic approaches, and the first two chapters can be skipped by those already familiar with these ideas and methods. The first chapter outlines the cognitive therapy of psychosis. I describe the model and the main intervention strategies that have been used. The second chapter outlines the psychoanalytic model of psychosis. I give a general introduction to psychodynamic way of working and go on to describe some of the alterations in psychodynamic technique that have been suggested in working with psychotic clients. I then discuss how some of these applications of psychodynamic therapy for psychosis can be used in cognitive therapy with psychotic clients. The remaining chapters describe the details of therapies of clients I have treated using a psychodynamically informed cognitive therapy. I hope that giving some detail on the clients demonstrates the great variety of presentations. In briefer descriptions, clients with similar symptoms can seem similar to each other, and their psychotic symptoms can seem divorced from other aspects of their lives. But this is the illusion of distance and has the unfortunate effect of dehumanising the clients by focusing on the symptoms without the context. The clients described in Part 2 have all been psychotic, and most have been given diagnoses of schizophrenia, but they are really a very disparate group. One important dimension along which they vary is the degree of withdrawal from the world into their own inner world. This relates to how socially withdrawn and handicapped they are. Some of these clients are working and have relationships and friends. Others are isolated and alone and incapable of working. Two of them are incapable of engaging in therapy.

The cases presented here have been altered in order to maintain the client's confidentiality following the suggestions of Clift (1986), Gabbard (2000), and Duffy (2010) and the method used by Lotterman (2015). I have omitted or altered personally identifying details. Furthermore, following White (2007) and Lysaker and Klion (2017), the cases presented here represent composites of several different clients so that, to some degree, these cases have been partly fictionalised. However, if clients gave permission for their stories to be included, the case has been altered to disguise the client's identity but is not a composite of several cases in this way. Where consent was given by the client they have read the relevant chapter before giving consent to its publication). I have not directly quoted clients' words, or my words to them, but I have paraphrased them (unless clients have given consent). In this process, I have been careful not to alter links between the personal history and the type of content that the client presented, but, following Lotterman, I haven't altered the type of psychotic symptom. So, if the client reports voices, I describe them as having voices, and if the client reports delusions, I report them as delusions. Furthermore, I haven't altered the theme of the content. So, for example, if the client reports derogatory voices, I have kept the voices as derogatory. In describing the client's social and domestic life, I have altered this so that it could not be recognised without altering the essential theme of any conflict either in the present or in the past.

There has been considerable controversy around "schizophrenia" as a diagnosis, due to problems not only with reliability and validity (Boyle, 1990; Read, 2018) but also on political grounds (Szasz, 1961; Laing, 1967). Diagnosing a client with "schizophrenia" has often carried the assumptions that (1) the cause of the problem is biological and that (2) this means that interventions should be biological. It does seem worth mentioning that it doesn't follow that, if the explanation is biological, this precludes psychological intervention or psychological understanding of the problem. The DSM and ICD-10 systems have certainly improved the reliability of the diagnosis of schizophrenia. But they constitute a list of symptoms from which the diagnosis can be given with by identifying a certain number of these symptoms, so that people can be given the label on the basis of disparate symptoms. If an underlying biological factor had been identified, it would be clearer where the boundaries of the disorder lay. One difficulty with using the term "psychotic" instead of "schizophrenia" is that some authors have made statements about "schizophrenia" and whatever was intended by that term it certainly wasn't supposed to mean all clients who are psychotic or who have been psychotic. If we replace "schizophrenia" by "psychotic", we end up misrepresenting what they said. When Kraepelin observed that the prognosis in dementia praecox was poor, he didn't mean that the prognosis for everyone who becomes psychotic was poor, for example.

One problem with the biological account is that it detracts from the psychological problems that the person presents with, for example trauma. Also, even if the reason why someone's distress results in psychotic phenomenon is because of their biology that would not mean that this explained what the distress was *about*. When, for example, Macbeth sees a dagger leading the way to the King's chamber in which he is about to commit Regicide, if the cause of the hallucination was a particular structure or chemical process in Macbeth's brain, this would not detract from the psychological significance of the hallucination (i.e. that it is Macbeth's conscience expressed as a sensory perception). And furthermore, in the case of Macbeth, we wouldn't feel that the most pertinent way to help him would be to alter the function of his brain in some way, even if this did result in the disappearance of Macbeth's auditory and visual hallucinations. It is an open question to what degree the voices and visions of those with chronic psychosis function a little like Macbeth's dagger. But I think that this is a different question to that of whether the tendency to hallucination or delusion or "schizophrenia" is inherited or caused by a brain function. If we wanted to explore the relation of dreams to a person's life, we wouldn't think that there was nothing to investigate if the tendency to dream was found to run in particular families and was more concordant in identical twins. As well as the cause of a state of mind, there is also the content of a psychological state, and how this content relates to the person's history and the person's life problems is not answered by investigations of their brain chemistry. Indeed, as Peter Strawson (1972) pointed out, we start looking for differences in peoples' brain chemistry once we have decided we can't understand them rather than the other way around. If we can understand someone's actions (or if we can understand the meaning of Macbeth's dagger), we don't go looking for a biological explanation. And sane experience, of course, is as determined by a biological process as an insane experience.

References

Boyle, M. (1990). *Schizophrenia: A scientific delusion?* London: Routledge.

Clift, M. (1986). Writing about psychiatric patients: Guidelines for case material. *Bulletin of the Menninger Clinic, 50*(6), 1–13.

Duffy, M. (2010, April). Writing about clients: Composite case material and its rationale. *Counselling and Values*, 135–153.

Gabbard, C. (2000). Disguise or consent: Problems and recommendations concerning the publication and presentation of clinical material. *International Journal of Psychoanalysis, 81*, 1071–1086.

Garrett, M. (2019). *Psychotherapy for psychosis: Integrating cognitive-behavioral and psychodynamic treatment.* New York: The Guildford Press.

Garrett, M., & Turkington, D. (2011). CBT for psychosis in a psychoanalytic frame. *Psychosis, 3*(1), 2–13.

Laing, R. (1967). *The politics of experience and the bird of paradise.* Harmondsworth: Penguin Books.

Lotterman, A. (2015). *Psychotherapy for people diagnosed with schizophrenia. Specific techniques*. London: Routledge.

Lysaker, P., & Klion, R. (2017). *Recovery, memory-making and severe mental illness comprehensive guide to metacognitive reflection and insight therapy*. New York: Routledge.

Nelson, H. (1997). *Cognitive therapy with schizophrenia a practice manual*. Cheltenham: Stanley Thornes.

Nelson, H. (2005). *Cognitive therapy with delusions and hallucinations*. Cheltenham: Stanley Thornes.

Read, J. (2018). Making sense of and responding sensibly to psychosis. *Journal of Humanistic Psychology*, *59*(5), 672–680.

Strawson, P. (1972). *Freedom and resentment and other essays*. London and New York: Routledge.

Szasz, T. (1961). *The myth of mental illness. Foundations of a theory of personal conduct*. New York: Harper and Row.

White, M. (2007). *Maps of narrative practice*. New York: W.W. Norton.

Part 1
Theories and Techniques

2 Cognitive Therapy for Psychosis

The Beginning of Cognitive Therapy of Psychosis (CBTp)

One of the ideas that led to the development of the cognitive therapy of psychosis was the information processing model of delusions. Jaspers (1913) had suggested that true delusions were different to other false beliefs in a number of ways. They couldn't be derived from any experiences and they were held with absolute conviction. He did think that some psychotic beliefs were derived from other abnormal experiences, but he called these "delusion-like beliefs". However, Maher (1984), an academic psychologist, suggested that delusions might be ordinary beliefs and that the oddness of the content of delusions was because they were ordinary explanations of abnormal experiences. A person hears a voice when no one is around and begins to believe that they are being spoken to by spirits. As well as experiences like hearing voices or having an intuition of reference, the person might have the experience that something strange or unusual was happening, and this more diffuse experience of strangeness can lead the person to come up with a delusional theory to explain this. A person has the feeling that something odd is going on. He or she begins to have the strong intuition that other people are reading his or her mind and begins to notice when other people look at him or her or when something he or she has been thinking about comes up in the news or in other people's conversation. These examples of reference seem to the client evidence that other people know what he or she is thinking about, and the processes of selective attention and confirmation bias lead to the strengthening of this belief.

The other main idea that contributed to the development of CBTp was Kingdon and Turkington's (1994, 2005) method of normalisation. They pointed out that talking to chronically psychotic clients from a medical frame of reference, about symptoms and illness tended to alienate the client and lead to a stand-off. They developed the method of talking to the client from the perspective of the dimensional view of psychotic symptoms and engaging the client in a conversation about whether the client's ideas were correct, rather than assuming that they were false. This proved a good way to engage clients in their own treatment.

DOI:10.4324/9781003168379-3

The hypothesis that delusions might be ordinary beliefs explaining the unordinary led to the attempt to alter delusions by using cognitive therapy (Watts et al., 1973; Kingdon & Turkington, 1991, 1994, 2005; Chadwick & Lowe, 1990). The information processing model of delusions leads to a goal of therapy being to alter a belief, which is a more attainable goal than the goal of "treating schizophrenia". Evidence that delusions seemed to be modifiable by rational disputation led to a renewed interest in psychotherapy with clients with psychosis, and this led to the boom in cognitive therapy for psychosis in the 1990s.

Cognitive Therapy of Psychosis (CBTp)

The Basic Model

If the client has had a delusion for many years, we can often be more certain about the factors that maintain the delusion rather than those that were involved in setting the delusion up in the first place. Sometimes, the client can marshal systematic current evidence; at other times, the client will really simply report a strong sense of conviction that the belief is true. If we look at this from the client's perspective, this (not being able to produce evidence for a strongly held belief) isn't as odd as we might initially feel. After all, if we were asked how we know our name is our name, we might find it difficult to come up with evidence. Other people generally know our name because we have told them what it is. Nelson (1997, 2005), Kingdon and Turkington (1994, 2005), and Chadwick and colleagues (1996) have developed ingenious ways of engaging with clients to test the validity of these delusional beliefs. These methods include modifying the delusion itself and modifying beliefs that maintain the delusion. Before trying to modify a delusion, Nelson (1997) assesses the implications for the client of the delusional belief turning out to be wrong. If a client believes that if he or she was delusional that this would mean that he or she was completely unable to have a happy life or that no one would want to know them, this would motivate the client to hold on to the delusion. Beliefs relating to stigma and hopelessness can also be targeted using normalisation and cognitive challenging. There are quite common non-psychotic beliefs which support delusions. That is, beliefs motivate that the client's resistance to changing the belief. (This is really somewhat similar to Garrett's [2019] ideas about working on non-psychotic defences in psychosis [see later].) Nelson suggests that beliefs about the meaning of being psychotic or having been out of touch with reality, or having had a mental illness, can motivate the person to maintain a delusion; consequently, she asks about underlying supportive beliefs before beginning to try to address whether the delusion is true or false. One important part of this is to have an acceptable alternative hypothesis about why the person has been deluded. For some people, the idea that they may have had a mental illness is acceptable as an alternative, and if the person already believes this, this helps. However, if this is not acceptable to the person, an acceptable alternative has to be arrived at. Normalisation of psychotic symptoms (Kingdon & Turkington, 2005) is a central part of this dialogue. Suggesting that psychotic symptoms, or having been psychotic, are on a continuum with non-psychotic experiences is central here.

There are a number of things about cognitive therapy of delusions that are quite different from cognitive therapy with clients with anxiety, depression, or personality disorders. How to cognitively challenge the beliefs, oddly, isn't one of these factors. One of the principal differences is in the process of engagement of the client. Psychotic clients often don't believe that they are psychotic and will have had many disagreements with people about this, some of which may have ended up with them being hospitalised or medicated against their will. In addition to these perceived negative outcomes, they are often very sensitive about being told that they are mentally ill. Not wanting to accept these negative outcomes, unfortunately, will often strengthen his or her motivation to maintain the delusional beliefs. To not want to be psychotic is, in itself, easy to understand, given the stigma around the label and the frightening implications of not being able to trust one's judgement about what is real. At the beginning, the aim has to be to develop a strong relationship with the client, and this means avoiding getting into an argument about whether they are psychotic or not. The universal practice is to avoid contradicting the delusion. A number of suggestions have been made about how to successfully engage a client in cognitive therapy. In addition to not arguing about the delusion, it is important to listen to the person's account of what has been going on and being interested and empathic about this. It is important that the therapist does not act in a way which confirms that the delusion is true. There are many situations in life in which we believe that someone else is wrong about some issue, but we often don't tell them this directly, for reason of tact and to maintain a good relationship with the person. If, to take one of Hazel Nelsons' examples, a friend has a new partner who we don't have a good opinion of, and asks us if we like them, we will often find ways to avoid the question, or we might lie in order to not do greater harm by upsetting and alienating them. Not being in the role of a case manager is important here. If you are the case manager, you have to intervene in the client's life in a number of reality-based ways. Is the client taking their prescribed medication, for example? Are they at risk of self-harm? You may have to relate to other members of the client's family who will have their own worries. And the client may have no option but to see you, so it may be a mandatory relationship, which again does not help to engage a client in cognitive therapy. Cognitive therapy is a collaborative relationship, and that is part of how it is helpful. Clarifying the problems from the point of view of the client is important. Some clients' lives are defined by their delusional system, so that they talk and think about little else; other clients have delusions or other psychotic symptoms but are bothered by other things as well. Sandra, who is discussed in Chapter 5, hardly ever brought up her psychotic symptoms. Other clients are consumed by their delusions and will want to get an assurance that the therapist believes that the delusions are true. I have found that most clients will be happy if you don't actively contradict them, despite eventually working out that you don't agree with them. To improve engagement at the beginning of the therapy, if possible, it is best to focus on something other than whether the client is right or wrong about the delusion: for example, discussing the impact on him or her of the delusion or, alternatively, discussing any other problems (if they bring any other problems along). It may be that the client doesn't see the delusion as a problem worth addressing, because what can a psychologist do about a conspiracy involving the government? (In fact, it is an interesting fact that many clients who are unshakeably certain that their delusion is true will want to talk about this with a psychologist rather than a policeman.)

As cognitive therapy is collaborative, if the client doesn't see the delusion as leading to problems (e.g. fear, misery, and social avoidance), it won't be addressed in therapy. Chadwick and colleagues (1996) begin by establishing a relationship with the client and then, after some time, suggest that it might be worth investigating the truth of the delusion because of the various negative consequences of the belief from the client's perspective. For example, one client believed that she was being monitored by the Echelon spy satellite system which, she believed, was watching her through spy cameras. The therapist suggested that, as this belief made her feel suspicious and made it difficult for her to leave the house, it might be worth checking if this belief was correct. If she was wrong about being spied on by satellites, there were many ways in which her life would become more rewarding. However, she felt that, if she had been wrong about this for the last 20 years, she would feel so devastated at the waste of her life worrying about this that she would want to kill herself. So, obviously, the therapist didn't pursue the issue. Hazel Nelson suggests introducing the possibility of the delusion being false in a gentle, hypothetical way and backing off if the client seems to resist going down that path. In Chadwick's later book (2006), modifying delusions is no longer necessarily the goal of the therapy. It is one possibility, if the client is open to doing that, but if the client is not interested in examining the truth or falsity of the delusion, he suggests that one should work on other issues, which seems very sensible. This might be the clients' negative beliefs about themselves, or about others or negative beliefs about how they are with others, or using mindfulness to help the client cope with their symptoms and with other problems, depending on what the client sees a point in working on. What is characteristic of all of these approaches is the thoroughgoing collaborative nature of the enterprise, similar to a solution–focused approach (Rhodes & Jakes, 2009). The client is invited to consider whether the delusion is true or not. This may be one of the reasons why the therapy is helpful, as often a medical approach deteriorates into a power struggle about whether the health professional or the client is right. Having a negative identity imposed is also damaging to the self-esteem of the client as well as being very isolating. Usually, a deluded client finds himself or herself alone in a world where other people invalidate many of the ideas that he or she feels concerned about, and where others want to impose a label on the client of being sick.

Clients are usually not very good at carrying out homework, so the therapy is usually carried out in the office. In clinical trials, the length of therapy is often a couple of months and the NICE guidelines are for 12 sessions, but this may be an artefact of the difficulties in carrying out clinical trials over a long period of time. Nelson sees clients for about a year, which is really more realistic. No one thinks that this is a curative therapy. The aim is rehabilitative. Although the evidence about the effectiveness of the approach is mixed, clients in cognitive therapy improve on a number of ratings more than clients in treatment as usual. Sometimes it has been hard to demonstrate that cognitive therapy is superior to more generic counselling, and it may be that the non-specific parts of cognitive therapy have a positive effect (Jones et al., 2018). One of the most promising things about the therapy is the demonstration that collaborative psychological therapy is well accepted by some psychotic clients, provided one makes the necessary adjustments to the approach.

Social Rank Model

Byrne and colleagues (Byrne et al., 2006) have developed a way of working with auditory hallucinations which addresses what they call the "social rank" implications of the experience. They point out that people with auditory hallucinations develop a relationship with the voice. The voices are personified and the person has a relationship with the voice (incidentally this might suggest that the phenomenon is more complicated than a misinterpreted abnormal perception). Usually (although not always), the voice is experienced as *powerful* and *bad*. For example, the client is often the weak victim and the voice is the strong persecutor. On other occasions, the voice can be positive and encouraging, or give what the client perceives as helpful advice. They point out that it need not have been the case that the client should relate to the voices in this way. Personifying the voice does not necessarily follow from hearing a voice. Of course, this does seem like a very natural outcome given that, in almost all other situations when we hear a voice, we hear it as the voice of a person. They have developed a refinement of cognitive therapy for psychosis which addresses this relationship to the voices and tries to help the client to reduce the feeling of being out of control and powerless. It is worth pointing out that this is a quite different theory to that of the information processing model. The beliefs about the voice and relationship to the client are addressed. How powerful is the voice? What happens if the client stands up to or ignores the voice? In the earlier, straightforwardly information processing, version of cognitive therapy for psychosis, voices have typically been dealt with by working on associated delusional beliefs, or by teaching coping skills. (I had a client who saw visions of people or spirits at the bottom of his bed every night. He believed that these visions were ghosts which had come to see him with malevolent intent. This was not part of an elaborated delusional system, although he certainly had other problems. My intervention with him consisted of testing the belief that the visions were actually ghosts or spirits which proved a simple exercise and altered his belief in the existence of the spirits in a couple of sessions. This is, in my experience, the exception rather than the rule.) However, in Birchwood and colleagues' intervention (Byrne et al., 2006), the client's relationship to the voice is targeted. This is done by identifying the client's beliefs about his or her relationship to the voice or voices and challenging these beliefs. For example, if the client believes that the voice is all powerful, experiments can be set up to test this belief. Often the therapist will challenge the voice to harm him or her, and when the voice doesn't do this, this is a disconfirmation of the belief. As well as challenging the client's beliefs about the voices, the therapy includes some role-playing exercises. The client is asked to dialogue with an empty chair in which the client imagines that the critical voice is sitting. An empty chair is placed in front of the client and the client is asked to move to the empty chair and to speak to the client in the way that the voice usually does. The client then moves back into his or her original chair and talks to the voice. The client might ask the voice questions about why it is talking to him in this way and then move into the chair of the voice and speculate on what the motive of the voice might be. This technique can also be used to practice taking a different attitude to the voice; for example, if the client is in the role of abused victim and the voice is the powerful abuser, the client can practice standing up to the voice. Sometimes clients feel that the voices are justifiably punishing them for crimes or errors that they have committed in the past, and this can lead to a discussion with the therapist about the client's perceived guilt and the appropriateness of the punishment.

Coping Strategy Enhancement

One of the first attempts at carrying out a cognitive therapy with psychotic clients was to enhance the strategies that the client uses to cope with voices and other psychotic symptoms. Tarrier (1992) investigated the strategies that people with psychosis used to cope with their voices, and they found that clients used a number of strategies to cope. They suggested that some of the strategies were helpful, whereas other strategies were unhelpful. So, shouting back at a threatening voice might lead to the belief that, if he or she had not shouted back, they would have been harmed, thus confirming a delusional belief. They also distinguished between strategies which involved distracting from the voices and strategies that involved focusing on the voices—listening to the voices and trying to understand their "meaning". Coping Strategy Enhancement involves asking the client what they do to cope and encouraging them to use the strategies that they already use more often. It also involves some psychoeducation about other strategies people use to cope. Tarrier (1992) asked clients to role play coping with the voice in the room with the therapist role playing the voice. The support and reward of successful coping by the therapist's approval, attention, and concern may well be part of what is helpful in this method.

Coping strategies are usually versions of distraction or diversion, trying not to engage with the voice or trying to understand the meaning of the voice, rather than pushing it away. This technique isn't really based on a model of therapy. Or possibly it comes from a behavioural model where skills are taught and reinforced so that they become habits.

Solution-Focused Therapy

Rhodes and Jakes (2009) have suggested applying solution-focused techniques to client with psychosis. This can be a particularly helpful strategy for engaging clients with no insight or who have been sent to therapy by someone else. One aspect is regarding the client's goals in therapy as paramount. If the psychiatrist sent the person and they are coming because they felt they had to, getting the psychiatrist off the client's back might be the goal of the therapy.

Beyond these, different models' cognitive therapy for psychosis has developed on an empirical basis. It has proved possible to work collaboratively using cognitive therapy with some psychotic clients (identifying triggering situations for problematic emotions; exploring the meaning of these emotions; and developing a positive working alliance) so the whole range of CBT techniques are potentially helpful. Prior to the development of CBTp, some people argued that talking to these clients about their problems was a waste of time or possibly harmful. Experience has suggested that this is not the case (Jones et al., 2018).

Schema Therapy

Several authors have applied schema therapy techniques to clients with psychosis (Chadwick, 2006; Rhodes, 2022). As Schema Therapy is itself an integrative therapy, some of these techniques are derived from psychodynamic thinking: for example, the Gestalt technique, used in Schema therapy of asking the client to talk to a part of the self in an empty chair. This method is not just derived from Gestalt therapy (Perls et al., 1951), but it also relies on the idea of thinking of "the self" as consisting of several sub-personalities or "selves", derived from psychoanalysis. In schema therapy, these sub-selves are described as "Modes" (Young et al., 2003; Young & Lindemann, 1992). The modes are named, for example, "Critical Parent", "Abusive Parent", "Vulnerable Child", or "Detached Protector", and the client is coached to confront or comfort these different parts of the self.

In working with psychotic clients, Paul Chadwick has used the method of talking to a part of the self in an empty chair in a number of ways. The client can talk to a critical or negative part of themselves and by changing chairs so that they dialogue with the inner critic and set limits with it. This part of the person can be labelled the "Inner Critical Parent", but often the inner critic is far more critical and attacking than the client's actual mother or father. (This is why Klein [1975] talks of part objects. That is part of the person. Actually, she talks of the good and bad breast. I take it that this is because she wants to convey that the internal critic, or the projected-out inner critic, is derived from the negative parts of the person and that it is as if seen through the eyes of an infant where gradations of good and bad and the complex mixtures of good and bad that all real people are comprised of are simplified.) The client can talk to a critical voice or a character from a delusion. These practices are often equivalent in that the voice is often an externalisation of the inner critic.

Here the therapist is directive and encourages the client to engage in role playing of various types with the aim of generating a new experience, whereas the traditional psychodynamic therapist is following the clients' train of thoughts, trying to understand the deeper meaning in what the client brings, which is a very different technique. The idea of separate sub-personalities in psychosis is derived from psychodynamic thinking. Although the therapy techniques are very different, the model of the mind is derived from the idea of dissociated parts of the self, which is so central to the psychodynamic model. The psychodynamic model sees psychosis, amongst other things, as the disintegration of the personality, so that as well as different parts of the self (or alternately the existence of different sub-personalities), there is no awareness that these are parts of the same personality. The application of schema therapy to psychosis has involved addressing parts of the personality which the client knows are part of them but also parts of the personality that they don't recognise as being them. When Chadwick or Rhodes asks a client to talk to a part of themselves which believes that they are useless, this can be Schema Therapy as would be applied to anyone else. There is nothing distinctive about this. It would be the same if the client were not psychotic. When he applies the technique to voices, when the client doesn't accept that the voices are not real, this is a psychosis-specific therapy.

Metacognitive Reflection and Insight Therapy (MERIT)

Paul Lysaker and colleagues (Lysaker & Klion, 2017; DiMaggio & Lysaker, 2010; DeJong et al., 2016; DiMaggio & Lysaker, 2015; Hillis et al., 2015) have developed a form of brief psychotherapy of clients with schizophrenia called metacognitive reflection and insight therapy (MERIT). The expressed aim of the therapy, as the name suggests, is to improve the ability of the person with "schizophrenia" to reflect on their own and others' states of mind. This is targeting a symptom which has not been the focus of cognitive therapy for psychosis and which is at one higher level, so to speak. This difficulty with reading states of mind of oneself, or of other people, is used to explain hallucinatory voices, delusions, made feelings and ideas of reference. It is not part of the list of symptoms in ICD or DSM criteria for schizophrenia, but it supposedly explains these symptoms. The method that Lysaker and his colleagues use is a modification of psychodynamic therapy, rather than cognitive therapy. Sessions are used to reflect on and clarify the intentions and feelings of people in the stories the clients narrate. In particular, the therapist reflects on the client's perception of the state of mind of the therapist. Clients are encouraged to give examples of events from their lives and the therapist then reflects on these examples emphasising the states of mind of the various people in the stories. The therapist also reflects on the interpersonal process between the client and the therapist.

Summary of Cognitive Therapy Strategies

Conceptualisation and Engagement

Generally, in cognitive therapy, after the initial assessment, a conceptualisation is shared with the client, linking the presenting symptoms or problems to current situations using a functional analysis, to associated thoughts and feelings, and to the historical roots of the underlying beliefs and behavioural patterns. This is used to guide the treatment. Kingdon and Turkington (2005) aim to produce such a conceptualisation with clients with schizophrenia, describing thoughts, feelings, and behaviour patterns associated with current problems using normalisation to discuss this with the client. Nelson (2005) also produces a formulation, which is more focused on the evidence that the client has for his or her delusional beliefs, but she differs in sharing this conceptualisation late in the process. She will ask the client hypothetical questions to determine how acceptable alternative ways of thinking about their delusions are. Of course, for problems that the clients know they have, this process is the same as it would be for any other problem. The complexity comes when sharing the conceptualisation would constitute a challenge to the clients' delusional system or denial of being psychotic. This is where Kingdon and Turkington's technique of normalisation is particularly helpful.

Coping Strategy Enhancement

Tarrier (1992) developed a method of enhancing clients' strategies to cope with psychotic symptoms. He investigated the methods that clients use to cope and found that they did indeed use a variety of methods involving distraction and other methods which involved accepting the symptoms and finding meaning in the symptoms. He encourages clients to develop a repertoire of different coping skills and points out the possible negative effect of some coping methods. The method also involves practicing coping skills in the office with the therapist—for example, role playing a negative voice. Along similar lines, Romme and Escher (1993) examined strategies that psychotic people used to deal with voices. They found that there are many strategies that people use and that people who seemed to be able to make meaning out of the experience did better than those who were overwhelmed or only avoided. They carried out a study of voice hearers in the general population and held a conference for voice hearers, which was the beginning of the hearing voices network.

Normalisation

Normalisation is one of the first cognitive interventions for psychosis as developed by Kingdon and Turkington (1994). As psychiatrists with responsibility for a particular health district, they began to talk to their clients with the aim of normalising the experiences and beliefs that they had, rather than from a medical perspective. This made the client an active participant in the treatment and reduced stigma and fear by negotiating a way of thinking about the psychosis that allowed clients to collaborate with the treatment team. This has been used as an important part of modifying delusions as well as engaging clients in treatment altogether.

Delusion Modification

As used in clinical practice, this means targeting beliefs which cause distress to the client. This is done in a collaborative way. The advantages to the client of investigating if the beliefs are true are highlighted, and agreement is sought from the client that investigating the truth of the beliefs would be helpful. The process of challenging the delusion is very similar to challenging other unhelpful beliefs. A key element in the approach was to focus on keeping the relationship collaborative as a key strategy. This means avoiding contradicting the client about the delusion without colluding with the client. Hazel Nelson recommends suspending disbelief or, if that isn't possible, talking from the clients' frame of reference. On the other hand, the therapist will want to avoid colluding with the client's delusions, as we do not want to strengthen the delusion by backing it up. The client will be given an alternative explanation for the evidence that the client has for the delusion. The alternative is framed using normalisation of the experiences rather than being a biological explanation. The key here is what explanation is (1) acceptable to the client and also (2) will explain the evidence in a non-delusional way.

Modifying Supporting Beliefs

Hazel Nelson (2005) has stressed that delusions are supported by non-psychotic beliefs which are involved in maintaining the delusion. She stresses that it is important to assess such beliefs and attempt to modify them prior to attempting to modify the delusion. For example, a client might believe that, if a person has a psychotic breakdown, they are worth less as a person. Or they might believe that other people might regard a person who has a psychotic breakdown as worth less than other people. Or a person might believe that if someone had a psychotic breakdown, they would never recover and might as well kill themselves. Obviously this type of belief will motivate the client to not give up the delusion. These beliefs constitute emotional reasons for not giving up a delusion rather than logical reasons for not giving up a belief. Prior to attempting to modify a delusion, she suggests that these beliefs need to be assessed and then addressed. Talking about psychotic symptoms as (1) continuum and (2) as a response to stress are two ways to normalise symptoms.

Changing the Relationship to Voices

Birchwood and colleagues (Byrne et al., 2006) have addressed the relationship between the client and his or her voices. The client often feels bullied by the voices. The voices are often seen as powerful, controlling, and malevolent. They work on re-evaluating these beliefs. They role play talking to the voices in an empty chair. Partly this can lead to a changed idea of the motivation of the voices. But it is also an opportunity to stand up to the voices and set limits.

Schema Therapy

Chadwick (2006) and Rhodes (2022) have used schema therapy with psychotic clients. Chadwick has used role play not only with voices but also with critical parts of the self. He uses this to promote acceptance of the critical inner voice rather than to challenge it. With some clients, it is possible to use schema therapy as with any other client not to address symptoms but to attempt to alter underlying dysfunctional beliefs and ways of interacting with other people, and also ways of relating to oneself.

Solution-Focused Strategies

Solution-focused therapy has been applied as part of CBT with psychotic clients (Rhodes & Jakes, 2009). The focus on identifying goals that the client wants to work towards, converting talk about problems to talk about goals, and investigating the client's current solutions to these problems are all very helpful in engaging a client who is in denial and in avoiding an unhelpful disagreement about the problem. Essentially the therapist takes the client's definition of the problem, explores what the solution of the problem would be like and takes this as the goal, and then investigates what the client is already doing to move towards this goal.

Mindfulness and Acceptance

Chadwick (2006) has described the application of mindfulness meditation training to encourage acceptance of psychotic symptoms. He makes variations to the usual practice of meditation to make it more acceptable to clients who are tortured by voices. He does not leave clients sitting in silence for long periods. In this, this is similar to the use of mindfulness in DBT with borderline clients, where adaptations are made along similar lines.

References

Byrne, S., Birchwood, M., Trower, P. E., & Meaden, A. (2006). *Casebook of cognitive behaviour therapy for command hallucinations: A social rank theory approach*. London and New York: Routledge.

Chadwick, P. D. (2006). *Person-based cognitive therapy for distressing psychosis*. West Sussex and Malden, MA: John Wiley and Sons.

Chadwick, P. D., Birchwood, M., & Trower, P. (1996). *Cognitive therapy for delusions, voices and paranoia*. West Sussex: John Wiley and Sons.

Chadwick, P. D., & Lowe, C. F. (1990). Measurement and modification of delusional beliefs. *Journal of Consulting and Clinical Psychology, 58*(2), 225–232.

De Jong, S., Van Donkersgoed, R. J., Aleman, A., Van der Gaag, M., Wunderink, L., Arends, J., Lysaker, P. H., & Pijnenborg, M. (2016). Practical implications of meta-cognitively oriented psychotherapy: Findings form a pilot study. *Journal of Nervous and Mental Disorders, 204*(9), 713–716.

DiMaggio, G., & Lysaker, P. (Ed.). (2010). *Metacognition and severe adult mental disorders: From research to treatment*. London and New York: Routledge.

DiMaggio, G., & Lysaker, P. (2015). Metacognition and mentalizing in the psychotherapy of patients with psychosis and personality disorders. *Journal of Clinical Psychology, 71*, 117–124.

Garrett, M. (2019). *Psychotherapy for psychosis: Integrating cognitive-behavioral and psychodynamic treatment*. New York: The Guildford Press.

Hillis, J. D., Leonhardt, B. L., Vohs, J. L., Buck, K. D., Salvatore, G., Popolo, R., DiMaggio, G., & Lysaker, P. H. (2015). Metacognitive reflective and insight therapy for people in early phase of a schizophrenia spectrum disorder. *Journal of Clinical Psychology: In Session, 71*(2), 125–135.

Jaspers, K. (1913). *General psychopathology-volumes 1 and 2* (Trans. J. Hoenig & M. W. Hamilton). Baltimore, MD and London: John Hopkins University Press.

Jones, C., Hacker, D., Cormac, I., Xia, J., Meaden, A., & Irving, C. B. (2018). Cognitive behaviour therapy versus other psychosocial treatments for schizophrenia. *Cochrane Database of Systematic Reviews, 15*(11), 2018 Nov 15. CD008712.do1.

Kingdon, D. G., & Turkington, D. (1991). Preliminary report: The use of cognitive behavioural therapy and a normalising rationale in schizophrenia. *Journal of Nervous and Mental Disease, 179*, 207–211.

Kingdon, D. G., & Turkington, D. (1994). *Cognitive behaviour therapy of schizophrenia*. New York: Guilford Press.

Kingdon, D. G., & Turkington, D. (2005). *Cognitive therapy of schizophrenia*. New York: Guilford Press.

Klein, M. (1975). *The writings of Melanie Klein, Vol 3*. London: Hogarth.

Lysaker, P., and Klion, R. (2017). *Recovery, memory-making and severe mental illness comprehensive guide to metacognitive reflection and insight therapy*. New York: Routledge.

Maher, B. (1984). Anomalous experience and delusional thinking. In T. Oltmanns & B. Maher (Eds.), *Delusional beliefs*. New York: Wiley.

Nelson, H. (1997). *Cognitive therapy with schizophrenia a practice manual*. Cheltenham: Stanley Thornes.

Nelson, H. (2005). *Cognitive therapy with delusions and hallucinations*. Cheltenham: Stanley Thornes.

Perls, F., Hefferline, R., & Goodman, P. (1951). *Gestalt therapy: Excitement and growth in the human personality*. New York: Julian.

Rhodes, J. (2022). *Psychosis and the traumatised self*. London: Routledge.

Rhodes, J., & Jakes, S. C. (2009). *Narrative cognitive behavioural therapy for psychosis*. London: Routledge.

Romme, M., & Escher, S. (1993). *Accepting voices*. London: Mind.

Tarrier, N. (1992). Management and modification of residual psychotic symptoms. In M. Birchwood & N. Tarrier (Eds.), *Innovations in the psychological management of schizophrenia*. West Sussex and New York: Wiley-Blackwell.

Watts, F. N., Powell, E. G., & Austin, S. V. (1973). The modification of abnormal beliefs. *British Journal of Medical Psychology, 46*, 359–363.

Young, J. E., Klosko, J. S., & Weishaar, M. E. (2003). *Schema therapy: A practitioners guide*. New York: Guilford Press.

Young, J. E., & Lindemann, M. D. (1992). An integrative schema-focused model of personality disorders. *Journal of Cognitive Psychotherapy: An International Quarterly, 6*(1), 11–23.

3   The Psychoanalytic View of Psychosis

In this chapter, I will briefly outline the psychodynamic model of psychosis or schizophrenia.

The Psychodynamic Model of the Mind

Psychoanalysis began with a view of symptoms as being caused by the repression of unacceptable feelings or memories. Certain traumatic memories and associated feelings were unconscious. The therapy worked by giving insight into the repression, and this gave the client awareness of the feeling or memory. This resulted in an abreaction of the repressed feelings leading to the disappearance of the symptoms. In this model, there is already the beginning of a view of the mind as consisting of parts—one part of the mind actively preventing another part of the mind having awareness of a feeling or a memory.

Object Relations

The current psychoanalytic model of the mind is mainly based on the theory of "object relations". The theory is that personality develops by identification with the mother and other carers, that certain role patterns are internalised, and that these internalised patterns then function to affect subsequent relationships. It suggests that the self can be thought of as being composed of a number of sub-personalities, derived from these early experiences. Furthermore, these sub-personalities are associated with complementary inner representations of "the other". So, for example, an inner sub-self might be a victimised child and the associated inner object might be an inner depriving or rejecting mother. These inner sub-selves and inner objects relate to each other. These patterns play out with other people and in the person's relationship to themselves. So, for example the "inner rejecting other" relates to the "inner victimised child" by attacking it. Or the inner object can be projected into someone in the outer world, so that a person's partner or therapist can be experienced as an "external rejecting object". Or the direction of the relationship can be reversed, so the client takes the role of the rejecting or

DOI:10.4324/9781003168379-4

depriving person and directs this at his or her partner, or therapist or boss, because the person has internalised both ends of a relationship–couple.

Psychological symptoms are generated by a dysfunction in relating to others. To be happy is to be able to receive and to give love, and a failure to be able to do this leads to symptoms. This is caused by difficulties in relating to people. This dysfunctional way of relating to others is the result of disturbed internalised object-relationships. The person recreates the problematic relationships of the past by projecting depriving "objects" into others. For example, a person has a parent who is depriving and rejecting and then internalises the relationship of "depriving object to deprived and angry sub-self". When the person enters relationships, they project the depriving pole of this relationship into the other person and then re-experience being deprived and rejected, which they then once more internalise. Or they adopt the rejecting and depriving end of the relationship and project the deprived and vulnerable pole of the relationship into the other. The idea of projection is that it is not just a matter of misperception. It brings out these characteristics in the other person.

The idea of an "inner object" was developed originally by Freud (1933). He had already suggested that the self could be broken down into different sub-parts such as the superego, the self, and the id. In *Mourning and Melancholia* (Freud, 1917), he describes the psychological mechanism of depression. He writes that the precipitating event is usually a loss of a person and that the client avoids the loss psychologically by "introjecting", that is, by identifying with the lost person. He suggests that if one examines the complaints that the depressed person makes towards himself, it will be found that these complaints do not apply to the client but do apply to the person who has been lost. So, the person, unconsciously, has incorporated the lost person into the self and then attacks this inner version of the lost person with the complaints that legitimately apply to the lost other. The shadow of the object has fallen on the ego which has been moulded in the shape of the object like molten wax.

Freud originally got the idea of an "inner object", the "super-ego", from considering the voices heard by people which commented on their actions and judged them. He thought that the delusion of being watched was derived from the same phenomena. What if the voices that people with psychosis hear were an internal agency that is present in everyone? In which case, the psychotic client is, in a way, correct about the existence of the critical agency. So, he postulated a super-ego which sits in judgement of the self (Freud, 1933).

Projection is not a case of misperception, although this is certainly involved, but the central idea is that the person's projecting of a hostile force into other people has a real effect on the other person's behaviour. The person behaves towards others in a way which generates the hostile behaviour. As well as the hostile external force, there is also a wholly good external force. These two parts of the other person are kept apart by splitting; a process in which good characteristics are attributed to a different person to the bad characteristics. The good is kept separate from the bad in order that the badness does not contaminate the goodness. There is a fantasy of a wholly good mother and the bad depriving qualities of the mother are attributed to the other, bad mother. Thus, the self is made up of a number of partially dissociated sub-personalities.

Fairbairn's Object Relations

The most influential theory of object relations is the Kleinian model. But Fairbairn's model (1952) has some interesting differences. He was heavily influenced by Klein (1975) but did not believe in Klein's postulation of a "death instinct", gave up the libido theory, and drew the interesting distinction between infantile and mature dependence; infantile dependence is unconditional—mature dependence is a choice. At the time, these were radical changes and they were rejected by most other practicing analysts. Fairbairn describes six inner objects. Three of these are self-states. These are paired to the three different "other" states. He suggests that the three self-state objects are the libidinal ego relating to the exciting object, the anti-libidinal ego (the rebellious ego) relating to the rejecting object, and the central ego relating to the ideal object. These inner objects structure the client's relationship to other people. You don't find out that you have one of these inner objects by introspection and they are not memories or images. You discover that you have these inner objects in a relationship with other people where the relationship is acted out.

In therapy, the therapist tries to work out which of these three types of object relations are being enacted with a view to giving insight into this by describing it to the client and by enacting a different type of relationship. For Fairbairn, dissatisfaction in relation to the mother led to splitting between the Good mother and the Rejecting mother. He thought that frustrations and disappointments in early caring relationships could lead to a sense of futility and detachment from other people. This sense of futility is not a defence but rather a painful state that the person defends against, for instance, by developing paranoid ideas about others. Fundamentally, the person seeks to be loved and to love, and it is when the child senses that they are not loved (or that their love is not received) that splitting of the object and the self occurs. These states are not conscious; what gets repressed are not impulses but bad objects, or bad self-states.

These rather abstract theoretical ideas stand in need of examples of how they are used to give them meaning. The object relations model leads to a helpful way of analysing interactions between the therapist and client, and in thinking about the problems that clients bring along. Often a client will present with a problem in relating to other people in some way. Thinking of these problems in terms of what general pattern of object-relations is being acted out can inform the therapy.

An Example

Steiner (1989) gives an example of a woman who described her mother as being treated with contempt and distain by her father and also by her brother. The client had done well academically. The client became depressed after giving birth. Steiner suggests that the client had become depressed as having a baby had pushed her into an identification with her oppressed mother. The client had a deformed hand, and Steiner suggests that she regarded her femininity as a deformity that she was being dragged into. Prior to this, she had functioned with a superimposed identification with her father, but giving birth had made it impossible to deny her femaleness. One possibility for therapy would be to help her restore her defensive organisation, that is, to regain her identification with her father, which denied her femaleness. In a second session, Steiner describes how the client denigrated aspects of motherhood, as a way, she suggests of trying to regain her identification with her father. A deeper aim of longer-term therapy would be to help her change her internal world in which her inner mother is bullied by her inner father so that an identification with her femaleness did not entail an iden-tification with a bullied and humiliated mother. This example shows the re-emergence of a bad object which had been repressed by another pattern of object relations, which, however, entailed disavowing parts of reality, that is, the femininity of the client.

Cognitive Analytic Therapy

Anthony Ryle's cognitive analytic therapy (1997) describes some of these processes using a different vocabulary. His model of borderline personal-ity disorder describes "Multiple Self States". These self-states consist of a number of different "reciprocal roles". By "reciprocal role", he means that we learn different roles due to our experiences as children and that these roles are best described as consisting of paired complimentary roles. These are named by the client in consultation with the therapist, for example, Vic-tim to Persecutor. The idea is that we learn a role pair; we learn a type of relationship so that when we learn one pole, we also learn the other pole as a potential role. Other reciprocal role pairs include Abandoner-Abandoner. These reciprocal roles are similar to the analytic idea of internal objects. A client, who is discussed later, had a borderline presentation. I met her when she presented as having been kidnapped. She had actually had an affair which had ended up with her being badly treated by the man concerned. This particular role, victim to abusive persecutor, had played out throughout her life in almost all her relationships with men.

Ryle describes the phenomena described by the analysts as splitting, (with idealisation and denigration, so that people are described as either wholly good or positive and others as wholly bad or negative) using different terms. The analytic model suggests that this is done as a defensive move. The good and the bad are separated to stop the good from being destroyed by the bad. This can involve projecting out the good object into others so that I am completely bad but the good exists outside me. Or the reverse "I am completely good and the other person is completely bad", because the fear is that, if they are brought together, the bad will destroy the good. Ryle, however, argues that such splitting may not be defensive but may be the result simply of immaturity.

Psychoanalytic View of Psychosis

Fenichel (1945) summarises the psychoanalytic theory of "schizophrenia" as being a profound regression to a "narcissistic" state. There is a breakdown in the functioning of the ego. The ego serves to distinguish me from you, and reality from wish fulfilment and fantasy. What he means by this is that, in response to trauma, the person's mental functioning recurs to an early stage of childhood development in which the person doesn't differentiate between themselves and others, and therefore a breakdown in the self. That this is a historical account is obviously a hypothesis. The other part of this suggestion that the person is in a more primitive mental state regarding function as a description of the current situation. So, the person gives up his or her "objects". This is different from turning to fantasised figures or memories from childhood, which is said to occur in other psychological problems, for example in borderline states. The person with "schizophrenia" has given up on relating to objects altogether. According to Fenichel, some of the symptoms are direct expressions of the effect of this regression, whereas some are attempts at a restitution of contact with others. This is an important difference to neurotic symptoms, in which symptoms are thought of as defending against painful unacknowledged feelings. As part of this regression, the client becomes aware of content of the unconscious which is usually repressed. The direct symptoms of regression to a state where the self is not distinguished from others are fantasies of the destruction of the world or the delusion of being dead, depersonalisation, feelings of grandeur, and the changes to thinking and other extreme states of non-contact such as "hebephrenia" and "catatonia". Other schizophrenic symptoms are attempts at restoring emotional contact with others; Fantasies of saving the world, hallucinations (where the person attempts to re-establish contact with the world by substituting hallucination for perception) and delusions in which there is an attempt to recommence interactions with others (and which often contain anxiety inducing elements as these were part of what made the person withdraw from reality in the beginning).

Carl Jung (1935) was one of the first analysts to suggest that the unity of the human personality was a convenient illusion and that the personality was, in reality, composed of innumerable sub-personalities which not only had characteristics of their own but also acted with what seemed to be a will of their own. So, for example, I may wish to take a course of action, for example studying a particular book, but I am diverted from this by another sub-personality which doesn't want this and acts to prevent this action, and I find myself watching television instead. Jung had worked under Bleuler and had seen a large number of clients with "schizophrenia". These sub-personalities are unconscious, but he thought that, in psychosis, these sub-personalities became conscious and were experienced as visions and heard as voices. Thoughts and feelings or unconscious modes of relating to others could become conscious. Experiencing these as visions or auditory hallucinations involves concrete thinking, in that a way of thinking and feeling is experienced as a perception. Also, the person is aware of these constituent aspects of their personality that they were not aware of them as parts of their personality. And external reality is seen through the lens of these sub-personalities. Jung's ideas influenced the novelist Herman Hesse, and the mental crisis of the main character in Hesse's (1927) novel "Steppenwolf" describes this fragmentation, and is a good place to find Jung's theories dramatised in the context of a breakdown.

Norman Cameron (1943, 1959) elaborated the theory in the following way. As a result of some environmental stress, the person begins to regress, there is a breakdown of ego, and the person begins to project negative feelings of hate and aggression into the environment in a major way. The person feels surrounded by hostile forces from which he or she has no defence. This is accompanied not only by a social withdrawal from other people but also by a psychological withdrawal. The client regresses into a more primitive type of thinking. This means that the person begins to operate with primary process thinking, the thinking of dreams in which logic is not primary or not present and associations are made by superficial characteristics of objects rather than by more meaningful characteristics. Furthermore, the clients' thinking becomes less conceptual and more "concrete". A metaphor may be taken for a literal statement. So, the person's ability to reality test is altered.

As well as splitting and projecting of unwanted impulses or feelings, the client can also project out positive parts of the self (to keep them safe). This projection leads to a lack of clear boundary between me and the rest of the world. Hearing voices is an example of this. I perceive my thoughts as coming from outside of me. Christopher Bollas (2015) talks of this process leading to the unconscious perception that inanimate objects are alive so that the psychotic person has imbued the world with life and fears that, if it wakes up, it could harm him or her.

Following Freud, Cameron (1943, 1959) suggests that paranoid delusions result from the client trying to re-establish a link with other people. When he or she comes up with an explanation of what is happening (the delusion), this relieves anxiety. The development of a systematised delusion allows the client to form relationships again, albeit with figures of the imagination.

This explanation is obviously radically different from the explanation given by cognitive therapists of the development of delusions. The analytic model links the person's voices, their delusions thought disorder and lack of reality testing as part of one problem. Furthermore, the underlying problem is that there is a change in the functioning of the ego which the other symptoms result from. Hearing voices or having delusions is not the problem; it is the underlying psychological changes which produce these symptoms. One important difference is the idea that paranoid delusions, and voices, constitute an attempt at re-establishing a relationship with the world, in which case one could argue that attempts to cognitively challenge delusions might be harmful. However, there is fortunately no evidence that cognitive interventions of this type have any negative effect, and, of course, no one suggests that medications that reduce voices or delusions are untherapeutic.

References

Bollas, C. (2015). *When the sun bursts: The enigma of schizophrenia.* New Haven, CT: Yale University Press.

Cameron, N. (1943). The paranoid pseudo-community. *American Journal of Sociology, 49*(1), 32–38.

Cameron, N. (1959). The paranoid pseudo-community revisited. *American Journal of Sociology, 65*(1), 52–58.

Fairbairn, C. (1952). *Psychoanalytic studies of the personality.* London: Routledge.

Fenichel, O. (1945). *The psychoanalytic theory of neurosis.* London: Routledge and Kegan Paul.

Freud, S. (1917). Mourning and melancholia. In *The standard edition of the complete works of Sigmund Freud.* London: Hogarth.

Freud, S. (1933). *Introductory lectures on psychoanalysis: New series.* London: Penguin.

Hesse, H. (1927). *Steppenwolf.* Berlin: S. Fisher Verlag.

Jung, C. (1935). *The Tavistock lectures: The collected works of Carl Jung.* London: Tavistock.

Klein, M. (1975). *The writings of Melanie Klein, Vol. 3.* London: Hogarth.

Ryle, A. (1997). *Cognitive analytic therapy and borderline personality disorder. The model and the method.* Chichester: Wiley.

Steiner, D. (1989). The internal family and the facts of life. *Psychoanalytic Psychotherapy, 4*, 31–42.

4 Psychoanalytic Technique and Psychosis

Psychodynamic Technique

In this chapter, I will describe modifications to psychodynamic technique that have been developed to work with psychotic clients.

Some Aspects of the Psychodynamic Model Important to Technique

Three aspects of the psychodynamic model of the mind are particularly important in understanding psychodynamic technique—symbolism, associative thinking, and the transference.

Symbolism

Symptoms have a symbolic meaning. This is partly because the motive for the symptom is being hidden from the client and is therefore expressed in a hidden way. Freud also suggests that as well as our rational way of thinking about ourselves and the world, there is also an unconscious part of the mind in which thinking is not rational but is dominated by emotions, associations, and superficial similarities. For example, a client was worried about problems in her marriage which were not being resolved, and she had begun to feel that she was moving closer to leaving her husband. She dreamt that she was in a lift which was going up when she wanted to go down. She pushed the down button several times quite roughly. The lift ground to a halt and began to fall. This dream symbolises the conflict she was in between feeling frustrated in her marriage and being scared of leaving her husband and what might happen. This presents as a dream partly to disguise the conflict from the dreamer (although it didn't do this very well). It also expresses the conflict in a clear story. It is partly that this is the language of this unconscious part of the mind. So, delusions can function in this way like dreams. Maybe they partly disguise the conflict from the client, and maybe they express the conflict in the language of primary process, or do both.

DOI:10.4324/9781003168379-5

Associative Thinking

In psychodynamic therapy, the client should say whatever comes into his or her mind. The assumption is that underlying important feelings will influence the content of what the client says and it is then the job of the therapist to interpret this to the client. The therapist focuses mainly on listening and noticing links, avoidances, or jumps in what the client says.

Transference

Initially psychoanalysis involved the client, under hypnosis, being encouraged to recall the details of the circumstances in which the symptoms first arose, and this led to the recall of childhood traumas. When a client recalled and abreacted a particular early trauma, the symptoms would be resolved (as they had been maintained by the process that repressed the memory). At least that was the model and the hope. In his article "Remembering, Repeating and Working Through", Freud (1914) suggested that the client in therapy did not remember a past trauma but re-enacted it in the session. This he thought was explained by a very basic process which was not aimed at maximising pleasure or reducing pain, but just repeated traumatic patterns. This kind of repetition is easy to see in the lives of our clients, and of course in the lives of those around us. A client, for example, who had a domineering father may act out a power struggle. A client of mine entered therapy with a concern that he wasn't being as effective at work as he could be. Soon after the sessions began, however, he began a list of complaints about his father who, he said, had been unreliable and critical. His father had told him that he would never amount to anything. At the same time, his father had a weak character and had let down his mother in a number of important ways. He worried about whether she was safe with him.

In the sessions with me, he would ask me to give him strategies and solutions to his feelings of low mood or anxiety. I duly suggested a number of things, and he either didn't do them or found them ineffective. He started suggesting to me the ways in which I could help him more effectively. I felt increasingly frustrated with him and the process of therapy and eventually, after some months, he dropped out of therapy without coming to discuss this with me. Here he has acted out a power struggle with me and, in the transference, I represent his father.

The focus of psychodynamic therapy changed to analysing the repetition of the client's problem in his or her relation to the therapist. The aim of the therapist changed from trying to uncover memories about past trauma to understanding the repetition of the trauma in the present. Analysts differ on whether or not it is essential to move from analysing the transference to linking it to the past. Malan (1995) would have it that this is essential. Symington (1986) emphasises the importance of the emotional experience in the "here-and-now" with the therapist. In the case I described, the client was talking about his father but, unconsciously, one can argue, he was actually not talking about his father but about me. Certainly, he ended up accusing me (implicitly mainly) of letting him down, giving him suggestions that did not help or that were not worth carrying out. He told me that, in the country he was from, men were more violent with each other than in Australia, and I think he was implying that men in Australia were less masculine. When first exposed to these ideas, it can seem unlikely that a client talking about his difficult relationship with his father should be understood to really be talking about the therapist who he had only met a few weeks ago. However, psychodynamic therapists insist that bringing this issue up in relation to the therapist is the most helpful way to react to this type of presentation. It seems undoubtedly true that underlying concerns, worries, and hopes influence what we talk about. At least they do some of the time. So, a client, when asked to say whatever comes into their mind, might end up talking about things not only related to their pressing problems but also related to the person that they are talking to.

The Basic Setting for Psychodynamic Therapy

This method is still followed, by and large, today. The psychoanalyst should ask the client to say whatever enters his or her mind. The analyst does not direct what the client should talk about and does not ask any questions but pays equal attention to everything that the client says. The analyst refrains from giving any personal information about himself or herself, apart from answering the question of what type of therapy the client is having. This allows the development of a particular psychological state which is conducive to the development of transference. That the analyst by being a "blank slate" allows the client to project onto the characteristics which belong to people from the client's past. The aim is to set up a neutral relationship in which the therapist deliberately avoids giving reassurance or encouragement. This set up not only allows the development of a positive transference but also allows the development of a negative transference—that is, the development of strong negative feelings towards the therapist. In fact, the therapist will spend a fair amount of time pointing out that the client has disavowed negative feelings towards the therapist in session. As clients will tend to split the person that they are relating to into a good and a bad object, part of the "cure" is to point out that defence. This is to help the person develop a more realistic perception of the therapist.

This then is the basic psychodynamic setting for therapy. The therapist endeavours to pay attention to everything the client says and does equally. The therapist maintains a neutral attitude to the client and doesn't reveal personal information about themselves. The main intervention of the therapist is in the form of interpretations of the client's unconscious thoughts and feelings.

Psychotherapy and the Science of Psychodynamics

Many of the books about psychodynamic therapy are rather abstract and obscure, and there is a point of view that psychodynamic therapy needs to be learned through supervision and personal experience of therapy oneself. This makes it difficult to really understand what is being described. An exception is David Malan's (1995) very good introduction to psychodynamic therapy, in which he walks the reader through the basic tenants of psychotherapy using real-life examples of clients he had treated or clients of therapists that he has supervised. He describes a modified technique which he developed in particular for shorter term and less intensive psychotherapy in which clients were seen often once a week, rather than every day, as is the case in psychoanalysis. The technique is more active. He gives a simple example of the approach of a woman who was in therapy and related an episode of becoming depressed. He says that, in such a case, the first thing that is necessary is to take a history of the problem and to find out what exactly had been happening when the symptoms developed. The depression had begun on a weekend away with two friends, another woman and a man. The other two had got on very well and she felt on the outside and had fallen into a depressed mood with feelings of self-hatred. He then suggests that an interpretation might be that the woman was unable to face her feelings of jealousy that had arisen, so she had turned a blind eye to the feelings (a defence) and that this has produced the depression (the symptom). In this case, he links the symptom of depression to an unacknowledged hidden feeling, jealousy. The woman had been able to acknowledge the hitherto unacknowledged feeling of jealousy and to express her feelings about this, leading to a resolution of her depressed mood and the beginning of insight into how her avoidance of the feeling of jealousy led to an unhelpful response.

How does the therapist decide what to interpret? The aim of the interpretation is to put the client in touch with his or her feelings or thoughts which are outside awareness and to link these feelings to other situations and relationships that the client has experienced. Malan (1995) summarised this process with two triangles which are intended as an aid to the therapist in the process of interpretation.

One is the triangle of conflict and the other the triangle of person. The triangle of conflict involves (1) the symptom, (2) the defence, and (3) the hidden feeling or hidden impulse. He suggests that any interpretation can be described as linking the corners of the triangles. The therapist might link the symptom to the defence, or to the hidden feeling, or the hidden feeling to the symptom. In general, he recommends that the defence is interpreted before the hidden feeling. So, with the case described earlier, the therapist might suggest that he or she thought that the depression (the symptom) was present because the person was avoiding thinking (the defence) about the situation with the other woman for fear of something that might happen if she did (the hidden feeling). By making the link between the symptom (depression) and the defence (avoiding thinking about her feelings), the therapist can see how the client responds. The client might confirm the link and might go on to say something about her fear of her anger, for example.

The other triangle is the Triangle of Person. The corners of this triangle are present relationship, past relationship, and here-and-now (the relationship with the therapist). Here the link is made again between the corners of the triangle. In the case of the girl with depression in response to the holiday with the two friends, making the link between the symptom (depression) and the defence (turning a blind eye) led to her expressing the hidden feeling to her friends and a resolution of the depression. If the depression persisted, one might link the feeling of jealousy in the precipitating situation to the relationship with her parents. One might suggest that the current feeling was related to how she had felt when, for example, her sister was preferred over her by her mother or one might link the feeling of jealousy to something happening in her relationship with the therapist, for example how the client felt about the therapist having cancelled a session. How does one know if such a link is correct? Obviously, there are a number of different and incompatible hypotheses that could be made. The answer to this is that the response of the client is taken as a guide to the correctness of the interpretation. If the client goes on to expand on the interpretation or to share more, deeper feelings, then the interpretation is correct. If the interpretation is met with a lack of comprehension, then the interpretation was inappropriate. Either it was wrong or it was correct but made at the wrong time. The interpretations which are thought to be most helpful are those which are made in the here-and-now with the analyst.

The psychoanalytic method, then, involves a focus on the minute-by-minute interaction between the client and the therapist. Given that most of the interactions that are important are going on unconsciously, it is important to have a way of becoming aware of this, and one way of doing this is to discuss clients in supervision. Another technique is to write out the session in detail.

As the relationship with the client is the main vehicle for examining the client's problems, being open to what the client brings to the session rather than imposing a theoretical model on the client's symptoms is important. This makes sense as the therapist wants to understand what the client is bringing to therapy rather than imposing a model on the client. This aspect of the practice has a lot of promise for working with psychotic clients in a psychodynamically informed way

Fairbairn's View of Therapy

Malan thought that effective therapy depended upon the client gaining insight into the historical origins of a particular symptom or problematic behaviour pattern. So, remembering and getting in touch with feelings about an early trauma and the link between the transference and the origin of this problem in the client's relationship to his or her parents were the key. An alternative view (held for example by Fairbairn [1952] and Symington [1986]) is that the primary therapeutic ingredient of psychoanalysis was the relationship to the therapist. If the therapist can be a good object to the client, the pattern of symptoms and problem behaviour based on avoiding the bad object could be changed. Interpretation is less important than a changed experience in the therapy. "Good object" obviously doesn't mean "ideal object" but an "object" who is not persecutory or narcissistic and is appropriately caring.

Adapting the Treatment Model for Psychotic Clients

How could such an approach be used with clients who have psychosis? Freud thought that it couldn't be used with schizophrenic clients because they did not develop transference to the therapist. This has, however, been questioned. If the therapist is aware of the client's transference towards him or her and of his or her counter-transference, the therapist is more likely to be able to respond to the client in a positive and constructive way, hence being more able to be a "Good Object" for the client.

Hanna Segal (1950) thought that it was possible to carry out an unmodified psychoanalysis, but others have disagreed with this and have attempted to modify psychoanalysis to make it accessible to clients with psychotic conditions. Fenichel (1945), writing in the middle of the twentieth century, made a number of suggestions about how to modify psychoanalysis for psychotic clients. He acknowledges that people with this label are very different to each other and that it is quite possible that there are several different types of disorder being classified under the same category. The diagnosis is not even useful in determining prognosis, he says. He thought that, with many schizophrenic clients, psychodynamic therapy is not helpful, but that if it is attempted, certain modifications should be made to the method. Whereas, with a client with a non-psychotic disorder, unconscious wishes should be the subject of interpretation, a psychotic person is already aware of much of these feelings and it is not necessary to interpret this, rather one should interpret how he or she is ignoring reality. He says that a major difficulty in therapy is the tendency of the schizophrenic client to drop or avoid human relationships so that, at the beginning, it is best to avoid interpreting things and to focus on building a positive rapport with the client, developing a friendly relationship.

Keats and McGlashan (1985) and McGlashan (1984) suggest a number of modifications to the analytic technique for clients with psychosis. McGlashan at the time was the director of research at Chestnut Lodge, a psychiatric hospital which focused on psychoanalysis for schizophrenia. Clients were admitted for several years. They suggest that an important part of the technique of psychotherapy is the attitude towards the relationship between the therapist and client. The relationship is consistent and ongoing; the therapist will be available and will not suddenly give up on the therapy; the client is regarded as dealing with problems which are versions of those that everyone deals with; the therapist balances emotional closeness with distance, and is working to increase the client's autonomy; and the client's privacy is respected. Therapy is not time limited; the therapist has to remain optimistic without slipping into a "rescuer" mode, and expects to experience strong negative counter-transference. Technically the therapist needs to establish a relationship with the client. This involves a long period of engagement in which the main goal is to establish a reasonably trusting relationship. Following this, the next intervention is clarifying the client's experiences by (1) listening and observing (including the therapists emotional responses), (2) looking for meaning in the clients' psychotic experiences and beliefs by engaging with the emotion associated with these experiences rather than the content of the psychotic experiences itself, (3) discussing the clients' emotions in detail, (4) clarifying facts around particular experiences (e.g. what exactly is happening when a client reports a conspiracy), and (5) naming feelings and connecting to particular people. Next they emphasise tolerating transference and counter-transference feelings. This is central to all forms of psychodynamic therapy. Later in therapy, interpretation is used to promote insight into their projections and how this links to relationships in the past and present.

Here the therapy differs from that with non-psychotic clients by having a long initial phase focused on engagement and establishment of trust and after this a phase of promoting understanding feelings. Interpretations occur much later in therapy. And therapy occurs over five years or more. This makes sense in terms of working from where the client is and, as most psychotic clients have little insight into being unwell or into their psychotic symptoms, this makes sense. Also, as the primary problem of the psychotic client is hypothesised to be a profound withdrawal from other people, this is working on the primary underlying problem.

Lotterman's Suggestions

Lotterman (2015) suggests that the traditional psychodynamic technique (i.e. waiting for the client to engage the therapist and avoiding directing the conversation) works well for neurotic clients but that a different technique is need for the psychotic patient. In this, he is following Kohut (1971), who suggested that clients with borderline personality disorder needed a different technique as the traditional method did not work for them. For example, borderline clients needed to have limits set in the way in which they interacted with the psychoanalyst. He describes how to modify psychoanalysis to make it appropriate for people with schizophrenia. He argues that the technique which Freud had described for working with neurotic disorders was not appropriate for people with psychotic disorders and that this means that, rather than concluding that they are not treatable using psychoanalysis, we need to alter the psychoanalytic technique for them.

The Nature of Psychosis

Lotterman says that there are several important differences between psychosis and other disorders of the mind. These differences are not those which are part of the definition of psychosis. (1) The client has a reduced capacity for emotional attachment to other people. The client has relationships which are shallow and brittle and which can turn from positive to negative very quickly. (2) The client has a disturbance in awareness of emotion and the ability to regulate emotion. The client may become abusive or very passive. (3) The client has a disturbance in psychological boundaries in that the person finds it difficult to distinguish different experiences in the mind. By this, he means that the person confuses dreams and reality, images and perceptions. The person can't tell the real from the unreal. Certainly, the last of these categories is characteristic of psychosis. Probably it isn't used as a defining characteristic as it is difficult to operationalise. We can derive the reality testing criteria from the fact that the person has hallucinations and delusions, but the other criteria are not linked to the DSM or ICD criteria for schizophrenia. The first two criteria have been used in the description of clients with borderline personality disorder.

He says that the breakdown in psychological barriers has a number of important effects. The therapist needs to be more active. He suggests that it is necessary to balance listening and being more active with the client. Clients with schizophrenia, he suggests, are very sensitive to being intruded upon, so the balance is important, but if the client is behaving in a way which might threaten the therapy, it is important for the therapist to act. He talks about a client who was about to throw in his job. He intervened and urged the client not to do this. He suggested that the client had a desire to be looked after by his family and that throwing his job in would have negative impact on the part of the client who wanted to be independent of his family. He justifies making a suggestion to the client on the basis that, if he hadn't, the client would have resigned and then been unable to continue to come for therapy. If the client was not acting in a way that might damage therapy, he suggests being less intrusive and to hold off on interpreting psychotic phenomena as this can make the client more evasive and defensive. (This fits with David Malan's [1995] suggestion that an appropriate interpretation deepens the rapport between the therapist and client [judged by the client talking more deeply about his or her feelings].) Interpreting a delusion when the client has no understanding that it might be a delusion is very likely to alienate the client and is therefore to be avoided, he suggests. The therapist needs to be guided by the individual client's ability to receive particular interpretations.

He suggests that it is necessary to set limits to other forms of behaviour. He wants clients to be involved in other forms of therapy as well as psychotherapy and he puts limits on destructive behaviour from the client. One client wandered about the therapy room picking up objects and breaking some objects. He relocated therapy so that he could have a nurse in the room to enforce the ban on these behaviours.

Lotterman describes a series of different techniques that he uses to deal with problems which are particular to psychosis. Many of these techniques are addressing the issues of the lack of insight into psychotic symptoms.

Meaning

He suggests that it is helpful to approach the session with the client as if everything that they say is meaningful, rather than thinking that some of the client's psychotic symptoms might be biologically determined. He suggests this, I think, because of the ubiquitous nature of the biological theory of the symptoms.

Transference

Lotterman makes a distinction between the transference and the interpersonal relationship between the therapist and the client. He suggests that, with transference reactions, the reaction is really borrowed from a relationship from the past, from a figure from the person's childhood. However, the interpersonal relationship is reality based. This seems to be based on this work as a psychiatrist and that this involves him in having to intervene in the lives of the client in a realistic way. He might give advice or prescribe medication. The client's reaction to these issues is, he suggests, also important. It is not obvious, however in what this difference amounts to. In both cases, it is important to draw attention to ruptures in the therapy relationship, or idealisations of it. Lotterman suggests that focus on the transference is important with schizophrenic patients, as it is with all clients in psychotherapy. Certainly, many analysts would regard all the clients' emotional reactions to the therapist as transference whether or not they seem to derive from a particular person in the client's history.

Counter-transference

He suggests that monitoring the counter-transference is even more important with psychotic clients than it is with non-psychotic clients, particularly because the client with schizophrenia may be less likely to be aware of and to express their emotional responses, due to the massive splitting which schizophrenic clients engage. The process through which the client puts these feelings into the therapist is called projective identification. For example, the client's feelings of emptiness can be induced in the therapist so that the therapist feels that he or she cannot connect with the client or wonders if he or she is wasting his or her time. One schizophrenic client I was seeing (described in detail later) became so anxious in the sessions with me that he could only stay for 20 minutes and then would ask to leave, often due to hearing voices in the room. Sometimes he talked about his symptoms or his worries and fears, and sometimes he talked about things which were seemingly unrelated to anything to do with his problems. He had a long history of being seen in psychiatric services. I began to feel hopeless about the possibility of connecting with him or doing anything useful in our sessions, especially as the time was so brief. However, he didn't cancel and he continued to come. I think that his is an example of a client's feelings of hopelessness being projected into the therapist, or of emotional induction if you prefer. This mechanism is, needless to say, unconscious on the part of the client and the therapist so that reflection on the counter-transference, or discussion of it in a supervision group, is needed to raise awareness of the feeling so that it can be used in therapy to the benefit of the client. In the case of my client, I raised the issue of his feelings of hopelessness when this came up as related to what he was discussing, and he agreed that he did indeed feel hopeless about his situation.

Lotterman suggests bringing up the therapist's frustrations with the client in a direct way. The problem with this approach, for example being direct about the client behaving in a way that annoys the therapist, is that it risks the client feeling blamed by the therapist for the way that the therapist feels.

Discussing the Therapist's Emotional Response

Lotterman suggests that disclosure of the emotional response of the therapist is helpful for the client. He suggests that this models the appropriate expression of feeling. He feels that the therapist needs to be aware of which of his or her responses to the client are to do with his or her personal life and those that come from the client. Supervision is one way to work this out.

Object Definition

In the traditional method, the therapist does not want to give away information about his or her life, so that the client can see the therapist as a blank slate on which he or she can project his or her personal problematic relationship and feelings. Lotterman suggests that, with psychotic clients, the boundary between the mind of the client and the mind of the therapist may be unclear so that drawing boundaries in the client's behaviour helps to clarify the psychological boundary.

Naming

This technique consists of putting into words what the therapist surmises that the psychotic client feels. This is done by asking the client direct questions to clarify what is going through their mind when it is apparent that the client may be reacting emotionally to some situation, and to suggest a purpose to the emotional reaction.

Enlargement

This technique goes along with naming. The name is taken from enlarging in the process of photography. He intervenes by directing the client to the content of a particular piece of behaviour and essentially asking the client to think further about it or say what comes to mind. This is very similar to the suggestion to ask the client for associations related to parts of a dream (that is to ask what elements of a dream remind the client of). Naming and enlargement involve the therapist taking a more active role than that traditionally taken by the psychodynamic therapist, but both are aimed at increasing understanding.

Voices

Hallucinations are an example of the tendency of thought or feeling to become concretised and experienced a perception. One consequence is that these thoughts or feelings cannot be thought about or analysed. Emotions are turned into distorted perceptions of the world. This is one type of splitting and projection. The idea is experienced as a vision or voice and this is located outside of the person. This may still be a disturbing or terrifying experience, but it is not linked to memories or to other thoughts and feelings or to particular interpersonal problems. His technique is to use Naming and Enlargement to try to explore the meaning of these experiences. He points out that, of course, experiences can also be reported to unconsciously further other aims and goals of the client, so that understanding this is not a mechanical operation.

Thought Disorder

He also deals with thought disorder by Naming and Enlargement. If the client is talking about an issue and then diverts to talking about another, unrelated issue or if the client is talking in some other way which is not comprehensible, he interrupts and points out to the client that he cannot understand how the conversation got from one topic to another. He says that there can be a number of different explanations for this. It is possible that the client doesn't understand that the listener will not be able to follow the conversation due to, possibly, lack of empathy. In this case, it is helpful for the client to understand that they cannot be understood. Alternatively, it may be that the client doesn't want to be understood, and the motive is to keep a distance between the client and other people. The therapist will persist in trying to understand the possible link between the two.

Delusions

One factor in promoting delusional thinking is the massive denial of consensual reality, because of its unacceptable nature. The fantasies of the client are given more prominence because they are not held in check by experience of our normal everyday reality. He suggests not confronting the delusional belief directly but advises the therapist to think about the emotions associated with the delusion, and how these feelings link to other parts of the person's life. So, if a client is fearful that they are being conspired against at their workplace, one should be interested in other times and places where the client had felt fearful or conspired against. It is also useful to investigate the clients' understanding of other beliefs that they have that are not consistent with the delusion. So, if the client believed that little men lived in his head, the therapist might ask about how big the little men were, and how they would be able to get into his head if there are no openings big enough for the little men to climb in. Partly here he is working to instil some doubt in the client, and this line of conversation will be familiar to the cognitive therapist.

When the Sun Bursts

Christopher Bollas (2015) also suggests modifying the psychodynamic technique with clients with schizophrenia. However, his suggestions are less radical than those of Lotterman. He says that waiting for the client to bring thoughts or feelings to the session is unlikely to be helpful. He suggests that the therapist should bring topics of an emotionally neutral type to the sessions, such as what has been on the news or what has been happening in recent sports reports. These topics are suggested as examples of emotionally neutral things to discuss. He views the psychotic client as extremely wary about contact with another human being, so the topics suggested by the therapist are those that are unlikely to distress or threaten the client. Actively introducing a topic into the conversation does not seem particularly unusual in other forms of therapy, of course, but is a departure from the psychodynamic stance. Bollas does this in order to begin to establish some link between the client and the therapist.

He suggests that it is important to spend a lot of time listening to the client's "myths" about his or her life, but that at some point, it is possible to try to connect the client to their real interpersonal history rather than the delusional history. He sees "schizophrenia" or psychosis as a retreat from emotional contact with people, and the development of an alternative history is part of a delusional system that distances the person from other people, so that the reestablishment of the clients' real history is part of reconnecting the person to reality. I saw a client who believed that he had met people at a rock festival who had told him things about his future life which then eventuated, so that he thought he remembered being given information about his future. In addition, he believed that there was a conspiracy behind this predicting of the future. He continued to work and to have a relationship with his girlfriend and his family, although they all found his account of how he knew certain things would happen rather disturbing. In his case, this type of work involved asking him about what else was going on around this time in his life, and being interested in not just the problems he had then but also the things that were going well. It also involved talking with him about his childhood and what sort of child he had been.

Another important strategy, according to Bollas, is to listen to the client, and what the client feels about what is happening to them. This is particularly important when the client is feeling empty or dead. This is a particularly difficult feeling, he suggests, and the only real response to it is to listen to the client, and to try to empathise with this painful experience. Eventually, Bollas says, it is time to offer the client interpretations, but this is certainly not at the beginning of therapy. When he does start offering interpretations, these tend to be of what the client might feel about the therapist or how the client feels that the therapist is letting them down, rather than about the client's hostility, because this is less likely to generate paranoia in the client.

Addressing the events leading up to the first psychotic breakdown is, he thinks, of the utmost importance with clients who have recently become psychotic, because he feels that addressing the trauma while it is still current can reverse the psychotic process. When dealing with voices, he will encourage the client to ask the voices questions because, as the voices cannot answer, the therapist and the client are left wondering about the intent of the voices together.

He also stressed that allowing the client to narrate their life is, in itself, strengthening to the person's ego. The simple act of explaining how things have been from the position of the "I" makes the sense of being a unified agent of one's actions stronger. And according to the analytic hypothesis about psychosis, this breaking down of the sense of self is the essence of psychosis. By sense of self, I do not mean to imply a "sense". The sense of self is manifested in the plans we make and things we say and do. It isn't an additional "sense" or perception (feeling that it is an illusion created by the language we use).

His method with psychotic client is quite different to that used with non-psychotic clients, but in an opposite way to that of Lotterman. Whereas Lotterman becomes more directive, assertive, and demanding of the client in an effort to bend the therapy to the client's needs, Bollas changes the therapy but in the direction of following the client more closely rather than demanding that client should follow us.

Integrating CBT and Psychodynamic Therapy

Recently there has been an interest in integrating CBTp with psychodynamic therapy. After all, this type of integrative therapy has a long history with non-psychotic problems. Garrett (2019) and Garrett and Turkington

(2011) have described how psychodynamic formulation can add to the understanding of psychotic clients when carrying out CBT, and that CBT strategies can help the psychodynamic therapist to engage the psychotic client. Reiser et al. (2022) report a case study in which a client was given 200 sessions of cognitive therapy over a six-year period. The client demonstrated improvement in preoccupation with his delusions and improved scores in depression and anxiety. Furthermore, he demonstrated significant improvements in social engagement. They suggest that the therapy involved psychodynamic aspects of the therapy relationship in addition to the cognitive strategies used and that psychodynamic supervision of the case added to the therapy.

Garrett (2019) points out that clients with psychotic disorders are going to have need of further support after a course of cognitive therapy for psychosis. Initially he uses cognitive therapy to work on the symptoms of psychosis, delusions, voices, and thought disorder. Once this stage is completed, he moves on to working with the client in a psychodynamic way. Some of this work involves linking current difficulties with issues from the past. After a period of working with the client using cognitive therapy, Garrett will begin to work psychodynamically. He stresses that this is not necessarily two phases with one following the other, and sometimes he will move back and forth between these stages. He will try to understand the meaning of the client's delusions. Usually, the client's affirmation of a link or a deepening of rapport is taken as confirmation of the link in terms of the precipitating events and also by looking at the client's delusion as a symbol or metaphor. The therapist can also ask the client what the delusional ideas remind the client of. A number of different interpretations of a delusion are clearly possible. Understanding the delusion as a metaphor or symbol is one way of thinking about the client psychodynamically. Also being interested in the detail of how the psychotic symptoms first emerged is a helpful strategy.

Garrett also talks about making interpretations of the non-psychotic defences employed by the psychotic person. There are a number of defences which maintain the delusional belief but which are not in themselves psychotic. Namely, (1) Refusing to accept that logic applies to them and (2) refusing to draw conclusions from a belief, thinking vaguely and simply restating the delusional belief. Also basing the belief on the feeling that it is true. These are, of course, familiar phenomena to anyone who has talked to delusional clients about their beliefs. In Garrett's model, they are motivated defence mechanisms to protect the delusion from being attacked. Actually, it could be argued that, in this, delusions are the same as other beliefs in which we are emotionally invested. These non-psychotic defences are a target for interpretation. This is very similar to Hazel Nelson's (2005) model in which there are supporting beliefs which need to be addressed prior to trying to modify the delusion. This is an important change from the classical method of working psychodynamically. The traditional aim is to not offer reassurance and to not aim at a "cure" but to pay attention evenly to everything that the client presents. It is establishing a place where the person can talk without aiming to try to satisfy the clients unmet needs even symbolically. Whereas in cognitive therapy, the aim is to develop a reality-based relationship in which the therapist and client work collaboratively to address certain agreed on goals by psychoeducation, functional analysis, and goal setting, with the prescription of homework for the client to carry out. If the therapist works cognitively and then moves to working psychodynamically, a particular kind of reality-based relationship will already have been established. Second, the way in which he works with clients is much more active than the traditional stance of the psychodynamic therapist. He adopts some of the methods described by Lotterman and actively confronts the client on issues about, for example, the delusion. Cognitive therapy usually avoids this type of confrontation on the basis that it can damage rapport and also that it can paradoxically reinforce a client's degree of belief in the delusion.

What Can Cognitive Therapy for Psychosis Gain From Psychodynamic Thinking?

There are a number of ways that Cognitive Therapy for psychosis can integrate some of these psychodynamic ideas. In a typical cognitive therapy of a psychotic client, the therapist may work on enhancing the client's coping skills, normalising the client's symptoms and work on modifying a client's delusion. They may also work on changing the client's relationship with the voice or voices. They may work on the client's self-esteem, possibly by encouraging a dialogue with a negative inner critic, or a negative outer critic (that is someone from the person's past or present life). They may encourage the client to use mindfulness to adopt an accepting attitude to the voices or the persecuting figures in the delusional story.

Most of the techniques and strategies that psychoanalysts have suggested as modifications of their technique for psychotic clients (Bollas, 2015; Lotterman, 2015) can readily be adopted by integrating a period of more non-directive counselling into the cognitive approach. Most of Lotterman's techniques are designed to elicit meaning from psychotic symptoms, whereas Bollas is mainly concerned with ways to temper the blank screen of the psychoanalyst so that it is more accessible to the paranoid client. Garrett (2019) and Garrett and Turkington (2011) have suggested working psychodynamically after an initial period of cognitive therapy.

Psychodynamic Conceptualisation

Conceptualising the client using the psychodynamic model is useful in a number of different ways. The client's symptoms and relationship problems are linked together. The symptoms can be seen as a development of difficulties in relating to others. Furthermore, these difficulties can often be traced back to early patterns of relating to other people. In this book, the cases presented demonstrate how particular symptoms can be linked to client's interpersonal problems in the present and in the past, and also how these difficulties can be related to the therapeutic relationship—transference and counter-transference. This model places clients' presenting problems in the frame of object relations. The client's internal world, the inner objects, and associated self-states are sketched out. Disturbance in these relationships is seen as leading to the symptoms and associated problems in present relationships. The evidence does not, in these cases, come from the client's affirmation of a link or interpretation, but from coherence as a criterion of truth. That is rather than a set of unrelated facts, there is a simplification. How we think about our clients is central to how we relate to them. One consequence of this type of conceptualisation is that the client is humanised. Biological explanations dehumanise the person, as do some information processing models. Psychosis is understood as an extreme form of splitting of the object and of the self. Identification is another important concept in understanding the clients' difficulties. This is related to the idea of internalisation of a particular type of object relationship. I may be identified with my critical and punishing father, for example. In a psychodynamic conceptualisation of psychosis, the client's symptoms relate to the client's history and the client's interpersonal problems. The symptoms are responses to these problems. This does not mean that there is not an organic component to some of the problems but the aim is to understand the symptoms psychologically. The client's account of the problems is the first source of information. The therapist listens to the story and observes what the client says and doesn't say and begins to think about possible links between different parts of the client's story.

For example, Sheila, a borderline client that I had been seeing for some time, had a psychotic breakdown in response to a breakdown in her marriage. I had been seeing her for a year and she reported that her only problem was her husband's outbursts of anger and controlling nature. They were in their late 20s. They worked together in a business that he owned, and most of the time, it was just the two of them. This meant that there was a lot of time to argue. His family did not accept her as she was not a Catholic. He got on well with her parents. They had been separated a year previously after she had had an affair during a break in their relationship. She was trying to work things out with her husband and they had moved back in together, but during a bad argument, he had pushed her and held her down and she had left him. This, she said had been a red line. She cancelled her next appointment implying that she was going to kill herself and then was admitted to hospital.

When she got out of hospital, she was brought to see me by her mother. She looked haunted and spoke with much more candour. In previous sessions, I had felt that the person with the problem was her husband and that she and I were getting together to fix him, and she held back on certain aspects of her history that might be embarrassing or show her in a negative light. She told me that she had had a psychotic breakdown. She had needed restraining and fought off the nurses who tried to hold her down. She had been hearing people asking her if she wanted to be killed and she had over-heard people talking about killing her. She had believed that there was a conspiracy against her and had dreamt about this too. By the time I saw her, these ideas had resolved. Her hallucinations were consistent with her fears in the recent trauma with her husband. Although she did not think that he wanted to kill her, he had harmed her through his violence and having to leave him had killed her dream of being happily married. An internal persecutory object was active in her psychosis and she felt pursued by mur-derous people. The boundary between her fear in fantasy and the outside world had broken and she experienced a fear in her mind as an event in the world. Another way of putting this is that her fear and grief get experi-enced as perceptions, turned into images, and then seen not as images but as objects in the world—here there is a link between the precipitating event (being physically harmed by her husband and realising that the marriage is hopeless) and the content of the hallucinations and delusions during her psychotic experience (a threat to kill her). The ideas have become concrete (she hears people saying that they will kill her rather than thinking about the end of her marriage)

The relationship here between the current interpersonal crisis that had precipitated the psychosis and the symptoms is clear. The symptoms also link to her personal history. She had had a number of similar relationships. The man she had had the affair with had contacted her friends and fam-ily and spread false information about her. In the past, she had had similar abusive relationships. She repeats the same sado-masochistic relationship partly, because she has internalised a persecutory object and a victimised sub-self.

The theme is also present in her childhood. There was no history of phys-ical or sexual abuse in her past. She described her mother as being a mild-mannered positive influence on the family. Her father was hot headed and critical both of her and of her mother. If we hypothesise that the original trauma dates to her relationship with her father, then her life demonstrates repetition compulsion. The initial trauma was her critical father who bullied her but also who bullied her mother. This is repeated in her relationships with men and, when she breaks down, is also repeated in her hallucinations of being threatened with being killed and, the delusion of the conspiracy to do this. It could be objected that this client is not typical of chronic psy-chotic clients, in that, being borderline, her hallucinations and delusions are linked to trauma whereas those of schizophrenic clients are not. However, the incidence of trauma in psychotic clients is very high, and if you listen to clients with a diagnosis of schizophrenia, they will usually talk about their trauma in a way which clearly links it to their history.

Sheila did not know why she kept ending up in relationships with men who abused her. When she had had the affair a year previously, the man she had been seeing had maliciously humiliated her. She had been rescued by her husband but then when her husband had later assaulted her and she had had to escape from him, she became suicidal and psychotic.

How did this play out in the transference? With me, she was very positive. Her initial sessions with me had been by phone and later by Zoom and the connection had been difficult. For some reason, she didn't have her own phone so that it was difficult to get in touch with her about the sessions. I really didn't get much of an idea about her in these first few sessions. It was much easier when she came in to see me and then a pattern was set up initially where she talked mainly about her husband's problems. She presented as being really well with the only problem being her husband's aggression and anger. I was idealised in a slightly distant way. Here one could hypothesise that the problem has been projected into her husband so that now her only problem is to fix him. This particular system continued for some time but eventually collapsed after she left him. Then the voices become the persecutors. I felt that I was in a position a little like her mother, benign but unable to confront the hostile forces that surrounded her. Idealisation is, of course, the other side of devaluation, so here there is the possibility that I will at some point become the abuser.

When she returned to therapy, she told me about some abusive situations that she had been in prior to coming to therapy. She had been attacked after meeting men that she had contacted online, and put herself in very risky situations. While her husband had been the problem in her life, she had not confided this in me so that this seemed like considerable progress that now she could share this.

Transference

Probably the most useful ideas that can be adopted from psychodynamic psychotherapy are the transference and the counter-transference. By transference, here I mean all of the attitudes both conscious and implicit that the client had towards the therapist. Often these ideas and feelings are implicit. Part of this involves repeated patterns of object relations. But this doesn't have to be a repeat of the relationship with a particular person. This idea is explored in all the cases described in this book. In a way, this means to turn one's attention away from the problems that the person describes in the world and think about the relevance of these ideas to the relationship to the therapist. Some of these attitudes may be very obvious or close to consciousness. The client may not say anything or may complain about some aspects of the therapy. At other times, this may be more implied. If a client shares something that they hadn't previously talked about, for example, this shows a change in the relationship to the therapist. Or the client might talk about his or her relationship to someone else. The client may, for example, mention how a previous psychologist had behaved towards them.

Counter-transference

Thinking about the reaction of the therapist to the client is also a key strategy that can be used in understanding psychotic clients. This is simply the other side of the repeated pattern of relationships. Sometimes this may be conscious or at other times not. One sign of this can be a loss of interest or focus on what the client is saying, or cancelling the client's appointments. In this book, I give examples in most of the cases. One example is becoming bored or sleepy or detached when with a client. Now, obviously, this may be explained by factors in the therapist's life. But there are some clients with whom we are more likely to become switched off. This can be seen as a re-enactment of a particular type of object relationship. Sometimes one can become aware that one is overly interested or disinterested, or angry or positive about a particular client. Being aware of these feelings in the counter-transference is useful (1) because it is an unconscious communication from the client and (2) because this makes it less likely that one will act this particular relationship out with the client. Some psychotic clients fill us with the sense of lack of connection. Supervision is one way to gain insight into these patterns.

Listening to the Client

Cognitive Therapy is a directive therapy, so this involves a change of stance. Bollas has suggested that analytic therapists hold back on interpretation to the client, but in CBT, this can be adopted as a more radical change, given that, in comparison to psychodynamic therapists, cognitive therapists are far more active in the session, setting agendas and defining problems. Allowing the client to tell his or her story to someone is, Bollas suggests, helpful as it strengthens the ego or central self. So that simply allowing the pace to change so that the client has the space to explain what has happened to them is a therapeutic strategy. If one usually wants to set goals and an agenda for change, this is a big shift. But allowing the client to narrate his or her story can have the power to change the story.

Connecting to the Person's Real Life

Delusions as narratives distance people from the real-life events that happened to them and the stresses that were associated with the beginning of the psychosis or delusion. There are several examples in the book of clients whose delusions became the only remaining social world, or even just a major part of it. Asking about what happened in the person's life at the beginning of the psychosis begins to reconnect the client to the real social world. This also begins the development of an alternative theory about the delusion. I saw a client who had a long-standing delusion that it was his destiny to discover a special new way of predicting the future, and that this would come to him in the form of a vision when he was in his mid–30s. When I asked what had been happening at the time that he had this realisation, it was that he had been in a long period of conflict with his father (of whom he only had negative things to say). His father had denigrated him for dropping out of school without passing his "A" levels, telling him that he was a useless failure, and he had developed this idea at that time. He said that his father had also been unfaithful to his mother, and in general spoke of his father in only negative terms. Talking about this with the client, without suggesting the obvious link, was a way of bringing him back to real but painful aspects of his life.

Taking What the Client Says as Having Meaning

Viewing what the client says as understandable in psychological terms rather than in biological terms is important in countering the tendency to objectify the client. This general assumption in most mental health teams is that the origin of psychotic experiences is organic and that there is no useful psychological explanation to be had, so treating what the person says as having meaning is quite a large step. This change in the attitude of the therapist is a little like the idea of suspending disbelief about a delusion or psychotic experience in that it is a change in the approach or attitude of the therapist rather than a change in the client. It seems helpful in that it counters a purely biological attitude, in which the therapist will not be connecting to what the client says or feels. Of course, we may not be able to understand the meaning of the symptoms or other behaviour.

Unconscious Communication

This is related to the previous strategy. What the client says may have implications that go beyond what the client deliberately intends. Indications that this is happening are when the client jumps quickly from one topic to another. So, it can be helpful to think about what the client talks about in relation to possible links between different topics or implied communications about events in the person's life, or communications about therapy or the therapist.

Thinking About the Symbolism of the Symptoms

If psychotic thinking involves concretisation, then trying to understand what the psychotic symptoms symbolise can help to translate these symptoms into abstract thought. In the case of the client who thought that he had a special purpose in life, this delusion symbolised his hope that he was worthwhile, being the opposite of his fear that he was worthless, as his father maintained.

Underlying Feelings of Futility and Misery

Bollas thinks that under the various psychotic symptoms are feelings of futility or despair and that all that can be done with this is to listen to these feelings and acknowledge them and that any attempt to problem-solving around these feelings will be unhelpful.

Naming and Extending

This involves the therapist thinking about what a symptom this might mean to the client and then suggesting this to the client. And then what this might relate to and what the client might feel about it. And then asking the client to say what this reminds them of or if it seems to relate to anything, A client, for example, might be hearing a voice telling them that they were useless. The therapist could wonder about whether the client felt other people didn't respect them and enlarge this by asking the client what that reminds them of. The therapist here is taking on some of the functions of the client's ego and modelling this for the client. With thought disorder, the therapist might ask the client how they got from one idea to another. A very similar technique is described by Kingdon and Turkington as a cognitive therapy technique (2005)

Probably the most important of these techniques is monitoring one's awareness of one's own feelings about the client and the client's feelings about the therapist. This can be done by monitoring one's feelings in the therapy room but is often better done by thinking about the session after it has finished. Trying to write out a transcript of the session can also help. The other way to become more aware of these feelings is by presenting the client in supervision.

Some of Lotterman's suggestions are not relevant for cognitive therapists (who are, for example, already quite active in therapy) but most could easily be applied, the therapy relationship in cognitive therapy being collaborative and the therapist presenting himself or herself in a realistic manner. His technique of naming and enlargement has some similarities to Kingdon and Turkington's method of working with thought disorder, explaining that the therapist doesn't understand how the client got from one idea to another. Targeting vaguer symptoms in therapy is worth including in cognitive work. The analytic idea that psychosis is generated by a regression to a more primitive type of thinking and away from social reality places the specific symptoms in a broader, albeit more sinister, context.

Thinking About How the Therapist Feels and Acts Towards the Client

As mentioned earlier, being aware of how one is feeling and acting towards the client is a central strategy. For example, being particularly keen to see a client or particularly dreading seeing client should give rise to wondering what it is about the client that gives rise to these feelings—similarly, finding oneself thinking about a client in terms of illness or feeling that they are beyond help. Alternatively finding oneself thinking about the client in the evenings or at the weekends may be another sign that the relationship needs to be thought about. Sometimes these feelings are clearer in actions. So, if we cancel a client's appointment or alternatively make a great effort not to cancel an appointment, this may point to negative or positive feelings that are being acted out in the session by the therapist, and this will point to behaviour that the client is enacting.

Beginnings and Breaks

Psychoanalytic technique draws attention to the meaning of breaks in treatment as significant interruptions to the therapy relationship which will likely have impact on the client. Of course, in psychoanalysis, the client is being seen each day so that a weekend break of two days may be felt as a definite change and a four-week holiday break will seem like a big change. If a client is being seen once a week or once a fortnight, a two-week holiday will not be so noticeable. The beginning and the end of each session can also trigger feelings of anxiety in clients, and that this is also true in psychotic clients will be demonstrated in the following chapters.

It is important, of course, that comments on these changes are thought about rather than mechanically doled out without thinking about the meaning for the particular client. Being given a ready-made link is not a very helpful experience.

Idealisation and Denigration

Often the stories that the client tells us either about their social world or about their delusional world will contain figures that are idealised or more often denigrated and seen as wholly bad. In these circumstances, it is often helpful to be aware of this as paranoid splitting, and to look for where the other part of the split object is located.

Often this will be in the therapist. Alternatively, if the client is idealising a figure, often the negative part of the object will be located in the therapist, but if not then it is useful to think about where the negative part is being located.

Other Important Considerations

How the client sees the therapist's view of the client is an important route into the client's negative feelings about themselves, so when this turns up it is useful to pursue it. How much is the client withdrawn? Does the client bring stories about interactions with others or is the client essentially alone?

It is likely that withdrawal from other people contributes to the client's progressive detachment from reality, so it is worth monitoring the degree to which this happens. Obviously, the therapist can directly observe the degree of withdrawal in the therapy session itself. Does the client bring feelings and anxieties to share? Is the client reassured by interaction with the therapist? That is, does the client let you into his or her world?

Content Related to Aggression

Psychodynamic theory postulates that symptoms of emotional disorder are defences against certain feelings or impulses, because these feelings or impulses are unacceptable. Often the unacceptable feeling is aggression or anger.

The Client's Negative Perception of the Therapist

Another helpful strategy is to be aware of the client's perception of the therapist. This can be a very useful way of addressing a paranoid response in a way that doesn't seem to the client as an attack. If the therapist thinks that the client harbours suspicions towards him or her, the therapist can take this up with the client, not in terms of the implied hostility in the client's view of the therapist but in terms of the client's perception of the client. For example, "You see me as a therapist who is keen to see you as flawed and damaged".

Transcending Theory

Another useful idea from psychoanalysis is that the therapist should not impose a particular theory on the client but should be open to alternative understanding of the client's problems, derived from the client's behaviour. Rather than imposing psychodynamic dogma on a client's experience, the therapist should be open to an understanding of the client's experiences which is novel and not summarised in previous ideas. This in part is about the sterile nature of imposing psychodynamic (or actually any other) model on the client as a procrustean bed, forcing the client's story into our idea of what it ought to be.

Levels of Interaction

In psychoanalysis, the therapist will wait for the client to begin the session and will not direct the course of the therapy session. Furthermore, the therapist will not disclose information about themselves. All this is in order that the transference is not affected by these factors and that the client is able to perceive the therapist purely on the basis of their past relationships and expectations about relationships. Often the client will deal with this situation by talking about his or her current problems, or alternatively the client may talk about the past (obviously there are other possibilities, such as silence but these are the most common responses). The therapist then listens to the client and makes observations (interpretative links) about what the client talks about. The aim of this is to help the client to be more fully aware of his or her feelings. In particular, the therapist will make links between what the client is talking about and the relationship in the here-and-now with the therapist. In cognitive therapy, the content of sessions is often to educate the client about psychological symptoms and to explain how these symptoms fit the cognitive model. Homework around the interpretations the client makes about various situations and setting up experimental tests of the client's beliefs about their, for example, delusional belief are important parts of the therapy. However, the relationship with the therapist will still have its ups and downs, even if the therapist imposes his or her agenda on the session or becomes didactic. Another reason for the dynamic therapist to not direct the session is that the therapist is clear that the client's reaction comes from them rather than being a response to a particular behaviour of the therapist. But as a matter of experience (see e.g. Ryle, 1997), these reactions are not abolished by the therapist setting agendas, challenging thoughts, and setting up experiments. Transference is everywhere.

Summary

Clients in cognitive therapy for psychosis can be readily conceptualised using a psychodynamic frame. This is based on (1) the content of the psychotic symptoms (what the voices say and the intention of the voices and what the delusional system is about). (2) The precipitating factors the meaning to the client of the conflicts which were around when the psychosis began. It is the meaning to the client that is important, of course although we are often able to accurately guess what this is. (3) The person's childhood experiences and developmental experiences through their adult life are also important. Having a detailed history of the client's life is helpful here. (4) Non-psychotic defences which perpetuate a delusional system are important. (5) The client's level of interacting with other people and, related to this, the degree to which the person's life is dominated by delusional ideas are important.

The client's relationship to the therapist is central to this formulation and the way that the therapist feels and behaves towards the client is particularly helpful. It may take some time before this is clear, although the initial reactions to the client are often informative. This formulation allows the psychotic symptoms to be seen as part of the person's overall psychology.

It is helpful to think of the symptoms as concretisation of particular feelings, conflicts, and memories. As well as symptoms such as hallucinations, delusions, thought disorder, and withdrawal from activities, there are also the softer changes to the psychology of the person with psychosis—for example difficulties in distinguishing between reality and fantasy or dreaming, which can be thought about.

Another aspect of psychoanalytic therapy which I have found particularly helpful as an addition to cognitive therapy is the use of the relationship with the therapist. The detailed interaction between the therapist and the client is examined as the way of working on the client's problems. This, of course, follows from the theory of the core problems being repeated in the transference, but whether one accepts this or not, it is a very useful way of dealing with the client's problems in the here-and-now, and in which there is no role-playing or acting about the issue (unlike for example in Gestalt or Schema Therapy). The detailed analysis of the interaction between the therapist and the client can be explored by reviewing transcripts of the individual sessions. The reaction of the client and of the therapist to the client informs this process. In the following chapters, I will give examples of the use of this type of reflection on the therapy relationship and also of using a psychodynamically influenced conceptualisation to add to the practice of cognitive therapy of psychosis.

There is a great emphasis on the here-and-now in psychodynamic therapy that can be easily adopted when using a cognitive approach. Presenting the fine details of therapy sessions with clients in supervision can help to understand these interactions in a way that can inform the therapy. In the following chapters of the book, I try to demonstrate how this can be used with psychotic clients.

References

Bollas, C. (2015). *When the sun bursts: The enigma of schizophrenia*. New Haven, CT: Yale University Press.

Fairbairn, C. (1952). *Psychoanalytic studies of the personality*. London: Routledge.

Fenichel, O. (1945). *The psychoanalytic theory of neurosis*. London: Routledge and Kegan Paul.

Freud, S. (1914). Remembering, repeating and working through. In *The standard edition of the complete works of Sigmund Freud*. London: Hogarth.

Garrett, M. (2019). *Psychotherapy for psychosis: Integrating cognitive-behavioral and psychodynamic treatment*. New York: The Guildford Press.

Garrett, M., & Turkington, D. (2011). CBT for psychosis in a psychoanalytic frame. *Psychosis*, *3*(1), 2–13.

Keats, C., & McGlashan, T. (1985). The intensive psychotherapy of schizophrenia. *Yale Journal of Biological Medicine*, *58*(3), 239–254.

Kingdon, D. G., & Turkington, D. (2005). *Cognitive therapy of schizophrenia*. New York: Guilford Press.

Kohut, H. (1971). *The analysis of the self*. New York: International Universities Press.

Lotterman, A. (2015). *Psychotherapy for people diagnosed with schizophrenia. Specific techniques*. London: Routledge.

Malan, D. (1995). *Individual psychotherapy and the science of psychodynamics*. London: Routledge.

McGlashan, T. (1984). The Chestnut lodge follow-up study. II. Longterm outcome of schizophrenia and the affective disorders. *Archives of General Psychiatry*, *41*(6), 586–601.

Nelson, H. (2005). *Cognitive therapy with delusions and hallucinations*. Cheltenham: Stanley Thornes.

Reiser, R., Turkington, D., & Garrett, M. (2022). Medication resistant psychosis: How many CBT sessions might be needed for recovery? A case report with psychodynamic commentary. *Psychosis*. DOI 10.1080/1/17522439.2022.2038255

Ryle, A. (1997). *Cognitive analytic therapy and borderline personality disorder. The model and the method*. Chichester: Wiley.

Segal, H. (1950). Some aspects of the psychoanalysis of a schizophrenic. *International Journal of Psychoanalysis*, 268–278.

Symington, N. (1986). *The analytic experience: Lectures from the Tavistock*. London: Free Association Books.

Part 2

Case Examples

5 Trevor and Kevin

Particular Difficulties in Engagement

Trevor

Complexities can arise in establishing a working alliance with the psychotic client. Trevor was referred to me by his GP for help with anxiety and I saw him at The District Psychology Service in Tunbridge Wells. He was 25 years old. His family contacted me prior to him attending for therapy. His wife told me that he wouldn't tell me the truth and that he was very suspicious of her. As I listened to her, I wondered whether she was overanxious or whether this was a sign that they had significant marital problems. I had rarely had someone's family contact me prior to the session of an adult client. As he had come from a South American background I wondered if possibly this was a cultural difference. His mother attended the session with him and insisted on coming into the office for the first interview. The first two sessions were a dialogue between Trevor and his mother with phone calls from his wife to me after the session. He engaged well and we clarified that he needed to come on his own. His mother said that she needed to come as he wouldn't be honest with me. We discussed this and I explained that usually therapy was the therapist and the client meeting privately and this allowed problems to be discussed in a more open way. She accepted this and we arranged that Trevor should come to the next meeting on his own. He arrived on time. He said that he had had some difficulties with anxiety, but these were really resolved now. I suggested we should meet for a few sessions to work out a treatment contract. At the next session, he explained that he had begun a new job. He was pleased about this. There were no difficulties at home. The other staff at work had, however, been a bit difficult. People had been making comments about him. Some direct and some indirect. He felt that they were making innuendos about his ethnic background and about his sexuality, implying he was homosexual. I discussed with him how he was dealing with these comments. He said that he didn't react, and I suggested that this was a very good thing. I listed the possible consequences of reacting, and he agreed. After he left, I didn't feel comfortable about his situation, all things considered. I wrote to the GP and the GP called and explained that he had seen a psychiatrist before, mainly about his

DOI:10.4324/9781003168379-7

drug use. She had tried to get him to take medication before, but this had failed. I contacted the mental health team. They said that they knew him from previous contact with the service and they visited him and carried out an assessment.

I got a phone call from his wife who explained that she wasn't sure if it was me that had called the mental health team but it had not helped. They had contacted him and had come around for an assessment. He felt that they weren't professional. Furthermore, one of the workers had been direct with him, telling him that they thought that he was paranoid. He had denied this. His girlfriend explained that he now believed that they were gangsters.

He later attended for his appointment with me. He explained that he had been well, and that the feelings that people were making comments or insults about him had gone. He mentioned that the team had come around and that they had been rude to him. He didn't think that they were professional and they were very young. I explained that I had called them as I thought that they might be able to help him. He said that he was doing well now and he didn't feel that he needed to come. I didn't believe him, but by this point, there was really nothing I could do about this as he now didn't trust me. All I could do was explain that he was welcome to come back at any time. This unfortunate set of events is a danger in working with psychotic clients, particularly if the client is seen in a psychology clinic or private practice. Because he was having paranoid thoughts about the other workers and having to restrain himself from reacting, it felt like an unstable situation. It was possible that he might react to a comment at work in a negative way, so I felt that I needed to involve the mental health team to ensure the safety of himself and the others at work. Unfortunately, this experience alienated him and he decided not to come back. Obviously, from his point of view, he had reason not to trust me. I had broken his confidence and called people to his house who he possibly believed were gangsters to come and intimidate him. This does not happen with every client who is not being seen by the mental health team, but it is a risk. If the person already has a team involved, then of course you never have to call them in. This incident demonstrates, I think, the effect of a paranoid delusion in alienating others and increasing the person's isolation. It is an example of the repetition of trauma. He came to me for help and ends up feeling that I have probably sent the gangsters around. Should I have called in the mental health team? A reason for not calling them is that it didn't help and that it alienated him from me so that he dropped out. On the other hand, if I hadn't called them then if something goes wrong, I can be seen to have not protected the client. If the client was involved in a conflict at work and I had told the mental health service about his paranoia, this could lead to more effective action to protect him and those around him. But I get pushed out of a therapeutic role and into the role of a policeman. It's much easier to work in a team, or with a client who is being supported by a team.

Kevin

Kevin was referred for help with his voices. He was a 40-year-old man who had a diagnosis of schizophrenia and lived at home with his parents. He was referred to the Dartford Psychological therapies department in Kent. He had had a psychotic breakdown in his mid-teens and had never worked and he had no friends. His daily routine would be a daily walk and helping his mother cook. He had considerable thought disorder, so that it was difficult to follow him. Often, he would say things that seemed to be contradictory, without being aware of this. His description of his childhood was very thin. He had a childlike manner in some way, but the main difficulty was that his reply to almost all questions was "I don't know" or "I'm not sure". I began by allowing him to talk and then trying to define some problems he would like to work on, but this didn't proceed very far. At first, I had found it very difficult to communicate with him. I mainly worked on trying to develop a rapport with him. I got the feeling that he was coming along mainly because he had been advised to by his psychiatrist and by his family.

I asked him how often he wanted to come and he had said about once every four weeks, so I arranged to see him monthly. After a couple of months, I got a message from his psychiatrist asking if I could see him more often and do some work with him on his voices. I discussed this with him in the next session, and he agreed to come more often. He said that he didn't remember how often he heard the voices and that he didn't think that they were a particular problem for him. Here his lack of an adult functioning self leads other people to pick up his goals and aims for him. The part of him that pursues goals or techniques to make his life better has been, if you like, projected into his psychiatrist.

After he had been coming for some months, he talked a little about his experiences. He did not know what to do about his previous psychiatrist, as he did not know whether she had been his lover or not. He also did not know if the voices he heard were real or hallucinations. This of course is a huge handicap for him. He couldn't distinguish between his imaginings, fears and hopes, and his memories. One advantage he had was that he was aware of this, so his strategy to cope with this was to be equivocal about most things. I asked him what he felt about coming to therapy and he said that he wasn't sure. As he lived at home with his family, he had as much contact with people as he wanted, and he helped his mother around the house with household tasks. He wasn't lonely. He had no sense of where he wanted his life to go, even in the short term. He trusted me enough to share some of his world with me, but after five months of attending once every three or four weeks, he stopped coming. I had asked him if he wanted to continue to come, and he hadn't known and he went away to think about it and never came back.

Here is a session near the end of therapy. He told me that the voices had bothered him about twice a week. He then amended this to twice every other week. The voices were there for about an hour when they came. The voices tell him that he has hurt someone or caused someone pain. I asked him if this was true and he said that it wasn't true. Did the voices remind him of anyone? He said that they reminded him of his relatives. He said that he was close to his immediate family but not with his other relatives. It was the other relatives that the voices were like. I asked him to tell me more about his voices. On previous occasions when I had asked him about his voices, he had said that he didn't know, or couldn't remember. In this session, he talked more openly about his experiences and beliefs. I thought that this was probably because not remembering was a strategy to avoid talking about his voices. I thought that it was probably a conscious strategy to avoid this topic rather than an unconscious defence, but that was also a possibility. Alternatively, not remembering could be a part of a disintegration in his sense of himself as a persisting person through time, and hence a sign of the disintegration of his ego.

In any case, talking more openly represented an increase in the degree of trust that the client had towards me. He went on to say that he saw the "voices" as well as hearing them. I asked him about this to try to clarify his experience. This was partly successful. He said that when he "saw" the voices, this experience was the same as seeing any other person. He said that the visions were not transparent or semi-transparent. They were, for example, recently sitting on the couch and talking to him. He had never tried to touch them. He said that he wasn't sure if they were real or if they came from him.

He said that he had a "spying problem". He said that he felt he was spied on in the street and at home. The voices spied on him in the toilet and in the shower. When he goes out on the street, he can see the people in the trees. I asked him if his parents could see the voices, and he said that they could. I asked him how he knew this and he said that he hadn't asked them and they didn't mention it but he could tell by the way in which they behaved when the "voices" were around. He went on to say that he knew his parents saw the voices because of the nightmares he had of people who tell him off and say that he is doing the wrong thing. I wasn't sure of the link between this and the voices that he had been talking about and it certainly didn't seem to rationalise why he believed that his parents believed that the voices were real or why his parents thought this. I asked him about the link and he said that he wasn't sure. I asked how the voices affected what he did in his life and he said that he was often not sure about whether he should go into the bathroom or toilet if they were there. At this point he looked off to the right and I asked him if he had heard a voice. He said that he hadn't and when I asked him about looking to the right, he explained that he did this as it helped him to think clearly.

In this session, Kevin told me much more about the voices and his beliefs about them. None the less a lot was left obscure. A technical difficulty here is that if one presses a client to explain the link between, for example, having nightmares and his parents seeing the voices that he hears, the client may confabulate an answer. That is, if we point out the irrationality of a particular logical jump, the client may fill in the gap for us, although they have never really considered this before. I think that Kevin had not really ever examined the links between his experiences and some of his beliefs about the world. Usually, I could understand what he was saying, but sometimes it wasn't clear what the sentence meant. In some ways if he had felt sure that the voices were real and not a product of his mind, things might have been more comfortable for him. Not knowing if his previous psychiatrist had been his lover made it very difficult for him to work out how to deal with the psychiatrist. If he had been convinced that she had been his lover, he might have had a number of emotional reactions, but he was often left in a limbo world where he wasn't sure what was real and what was imagination, including what he could see with his eyes. It meant that he never knew what was fantasy.

I thought an important part of this session was that he told me in more detail about these experiences and what he felt about them. It would be a mistake to be focused on reality testing these experiences at this stage, as it would be likely to discourage him from talking to me about these secrets. Probably in the past when he has talked to others about this, it has led to negative consequences.

What is happening in the transference and counter-transference in Kevin's case? It is hard to make an emotional connection to him because, for whatever reason, he responds to my questions with "I'm not sure" or "I don't remember". Also, he volunteers little about his past. There was no sense of anxiety or distress in the sessions. He was happy to be in the office with me. There again he would be happy not to be. Although his psychiatrist thought that he needed help with his voices, this topic only came up because I raised it with him, and if the voices distressed him, then it wasn't to the degree that he remembered it. Of course, an alternative hypothesis here is that he did remember the distress about the voices but was not sure that he wanted to let me in. The session I presented earlier, in which he did talk about some of his experiences, is consistent with the suggestion that he is holding back on talking about his experiences, at least to some degree.

What can be done here? Of all the clients presented, Kevin seems the most lost in his own internal world. He doesn't have a developed delusional system to explain what has happened to him. He can't distinguish between his memories and his fantasies to the extent that he doesn't know if his doctor had been his lover. Here the most important thing seems to see the client over a long period of time, in order to establish the therapist as a good object in a world in which his ability to determine what is his imagining and what is reality has reached the point that he thinks it wisest not to pass comment. Unfortunately, he dropped out. He didn't seem to be distressed about any of the things he told me about, and he wasn't particularly engaged in the process of coming. After all he chose to come once a month at the outset.

6 Sandra

Voices From Mars—A Delusion in the Background

Sandra was referred to me as one of the first patients that I saw in private practice. Her GP referred her for help in coping with her suicidal feelings. She had a diagnosis of schizophrenia. She was 40 years of age and was referred because she had been feeling suicidal. I saw her in a small clinic which was mainly used for physiotherapy and was actually a converted one-story house. She was in a long-term relationship with an older woman who had been a nurse in the army. They had been together for 20 years. Her partner was sick with heart failure. She had moved out and moved near to her mother. In the past, she had made a number of suicide attempts, and this was why the GP referred her, in all probability. She hadn't worked for many years and had no children. She had had several admissions to psychiatric hospitals and recently had been discharged after an admission to help her withdraw from benzodiazepines which she had become addicted to after having them prescribed by her psychiatrist.

She began by explaining that she was living between two houses and this was difficult. Her girlfriend Jane was increasingly unable to look after herself, but she had nurses coming in to see her. Sandra went back to cook for her. She didn't mention any psychotic symptoms and the main thing that she wanted help with was her low mood. She said that she had been feeling more depressed and anxious and that she was feeling overwhelmed. She had a difficult relationship with her mother. She remembered her mother as being quite cruel to her as a child. She also felt that her mother favoured her brothers as more important when she was a child and also now as adults. She never felt safe. Her mother would expect her to do things for her and would prioritise the needs and wishes of her brothers over hers in the present as well as in the past. This left her feeling both resentful and as if there was something wrong with her. She felt that she didn't fit in at school and she truanted a lot of the time, particularly in high school. A major trauma of her childhood was the sense of neglect and being treated as not really worth anything at all. She remembered her mother as being relentlessly critical and demanding of her. Her mother was unpredictably angry and Sandra often felt that she was physically punished

DOI:10.4324/9781003168379-8

for things outside her control. She remembers being given alcohol when she was in primary school. She always seemed to be not good enough or not doing the right thing. When she was around 8 years old, she was sexually abused by a family friend, and she wasn't able to talk to her parents about this.

Essentially, she felt that she had little value and that her family did not protect her and actively harmed her. The world was a dangerous place and there were no protective people looking out for her. She began to set fires and skip school. When she skipped school, she spent the time on her own as she had no friends.

I began by setting up an agreement that she would come for four sessions and then we could plan what we might do. She went on living across two houses for many months. From the beginning, she developed a positive, idealised transference. Many years later, she told me that she felt that she could trust me from the first session. During the initial sessions, I took a history and we agreed that we would meet to work on lifting her mood. I began working with her using behavioural activation, that is, encouraging her to timetable activities for the day. Really, she presented as a woman with depression who was trying to deal with the break-up of her relationship, and was struggling. And this was making her feel suicidal. Although I knew she had a diagnosis of schizophrenia, I wouldn't have known this from the problems that she presented. She felt overwhelmed by moving back and forth between her home with her partner and her mother's house, particularly as she had no car.

Shortly after therapy began, she rang me at home on a Sunday. I had said that if she felt unsafe, she could do this. She began talking in a rather vague way about how she was feeling but then it emerged from her description of the brightness of the water that she was actually standing on the edge of a cliff thinking about throwing herself off. She agreed to go home. Over the next few weeks, she mainly talked about feeling depressed and her problems with her partner. I had been seeing her once a fortnight for two months. As her thoughts of killing herself were actually quite often present, she was admitted to hospital for about six months. Shortly after this, she and her partner decided to end their relationship.

She had several workers who would help her with her shopping and going to various appointments. She has a dark sense of humour and she would laugh at people suggesting that she should go out to more activities. She said that she was already flat out going to various meetings with doctors and other appointments. She spent the days with her elderly, disabled mother and retreated in the evenings to her rented flat. She went to bed in the late afternoon. She used to watch TV and listen to music and she felt soothed by watching the same series all the time.

An important recent event was that she had lost her driving licence, as she had fallen asleep at the wheel and crossed the centre line and collided with a car head on. She remembered little of the accident but as she had been on high-dose prescribed diazepam at the time, she had resolved to stop taking it and had successfully done this. One of her aims was to get her licence back.

She found dealing with the crisis of her separation overwhelming. The house was sold and the proceeds from the sale were not enough to buy another house, so she ended up as a lodger in a house near to her mother. This was a difficult new beginning for her. I didn't really understand at the time how difficult her relationship with her mother had been.

At this point in the therapy, I had a client who had been continually reacting to crises. First, she had been coping with the separation from her partner on whom she had been financially dependent and, second, she had been admitted to hospital (which although it kept her safe also traumatised her), and third, she lost her home and was now in a dependant position of being a lodger. Her girlfriend had become dependent on her due to her illness and now her mother became dependant on her. So, the interpersonal theme here is the reversal of the nature of her primary current relationship. The relationship has changed from her being dependent and abused to having her partner and mother depend on her. After she had got out of hospital, she settled in to looking after her mother. This was particularly difficult for her. She had left home in her teens and had never felt that her mother had cared for her, and now she was in a position of being expected to care for her mother. Her memories of being a child were of being put down, blamed, and criticised, treated as if there was something wrong with her.

After three or four months of therapy, she began to tell me about her psychotic experiences. She didn't present these as particular problems for her or even as symptoms but they came up in conversation. She had visions of her dead father. She would see him in various places. When she saw him, she was afraid, but she couldn't really say of what she was afraid. She thought not only that this was a vision but also that it was not a vision and that he was really there. If I pointed out the contradiction, she would not be able to say how it could be the case. He didn't speak to her or touch her but he looked at her with an intense and unblinking gaze.

At another time, she said that she had always known that she had been born on Mars. It was clear that she meant this literally. She didn't have a complicated delusional system to explain how this had happened, but it had always been her belief and there was nothing metaphorical about it at all. She knew she was a Martian. There is, of course, nothing unusual in having a belief which you can't justify by reference to evidence. Many of our beliefs are held because we have learnt them from others (who we may believe can justify the belief). What is unusual and psychotic about this belief is that is idiosyncratic. This is a non-socially learnt belief. It's not that this belief is out of tune with the evidence, but that it is radically non-conformist that makes it psychotic. She also heard voices. Sometimes it was the voice of her ex-partner, sometimes it was her dead father and sometimes it was the voice of the Devil talking to her, saying "Kill yourself" or "You are rubbish". Sometimes when she was out in public, she was sure that other people could read her mind.

It is noteworthy that she did not connect any of her psychotic experiences to her life experiences, although for an outsider, it is not difficult to do. If these statements or experiences were connected to her other experiences, they might not be so clearly psychotic. Why does she not connect them? The psychodynamic model is that this is motivated. These experiences are split off, or dissociated from the life experiences to which they relate. This may be done to avoid fear and pain, or to prevent hostile or aggressive impulses from destroying each other. But it may also represent a disintegration of the integrative function of the self. (Of course, this does not imply that there are not other, possibly biological, factors which predispose someone to these types of reactions.)

Thinking of these experiences in this way will alter how we go about relating to them. If a belief is a way of keeping the person safe, that is has a function. If a belief demonstrates a regression to an unintegrated, primitive state of mind, it will be more of a description of a mental disaster. In either case, we will be less inclined to see challenging the belief as the primary purpose in therapy, whereas if a belief is simply a consequence, for example, of faulty information processing, altering the belief (if possible) would be a primary goal.

So, with Sandra, I didn't jump into challenging her delusions or beliefs about her being an alien or nature of her voices and visions. Partly this was not only because they weren't presented as the most pressing problem but also because it seemed more important to address the need that the delusion might be fulfilling, or if you like the "meaning" of the delusion, that is, what the delusion symbolised. In our sessions, I began by listening to her distress about losing her partner and looking after her mother, after having escaped this situation years before. She felt trapped.

She found her mother intensely irritating. Her mother was confined to a chair and couldn't walk alone. If Sandra left the house, she would ring her up to find out when she would be back. Her relationship with her mother had changed. The balance of power had reversed. Her mother no longer put her down continually. But Sandra still felt her mother put her brothers first. For example, at one point, Sandra was left with some money by an aunt and her mother insisted that she gave some of this to her brothers, even though Sandra was in need of the money to find her own place to live. She felt as if she were back in the situation she was in prior to leaving home in her teens. This feeling increased the irritation she felt when her mother called. She found visits to the house by her brother and his family very painful and tried as much as possible to avoid them.

My understanding of her history evolved over a considerable period of time, and at the beginning, I knew very little about her background. Because she was in crisis, I didn't take a detailed history in the usual way. It would have been better to have taken a comprehensive personal history, of course. However, even if one does, there are always important details about the persons past that he or she omits for various reasons. At this point, her story was far clearer. Whether this was because she related it in a clearer way, or because I was more receptive and attentive to what she said is open to debate. Probably the truth lies in-between. Her father had been always at work. When he was around, he had been critical and controlling. Her mother was always critical and abusive. She remembered being chased around the garden by her mother when she was about 4 or 5 years old with her mother trying to hit her with a frying pan. Her father in response to this had cut a leather strap to hit Sandra with. A family friend was sexually abusing her from about the age of 8. She truanted from school and set fires. She took pleasure in being defiant at school. No one seems to have wondered why. She said that she heard voices from the age of 5 and thought that everyone else heard voices. I have had several clients who have independently reported hearing voices from childhood. There seems no reason to doubt her account. She left home as early as she could, around the age of 15 and got work as a nursing assistant. She shared a flat with a male friend, but he always had friends around who smoked grass so she asked him to leave and lived alone. Sometimes she lived on cornflakes as she didn't have much money left after she paid the rent. But she was used to that.

She was always interested in older men. She thought that this was because she was looking for a father figure. Boys of her age never interested her. She had an affair with a married man. It was part of the attraction that he was already involved with someone else and wouldn't make any demands on her. When she finally met her partner, she was a woman of twice her age. They began dating and then they moved in together. Her partner was a more senior nurse. She described her as controlling and critical. She used to want to know where Sandra was going and with whom. Later she called Sandra a "mad cow". She gave up her nursing job to look after Sandra, so then it was just the two of them. Here is an example of the compulsion to repeat in her life outside of therapy. She fled from a home where she felt uncared for and criticised and abused and she ended up in a relationship with an older woman which repeats most of these characteristics. Freud thought that the compulsion to repeat was not derived from an attempt to achieve pleasure but was a more primitive process without a further aim. Fairbairn, on the other hand, thought that this was just the return of a repressed bad internal object—that if a person has internalised a persecuting object, they will repress it but it will continue to return in the relationships that they have.

After this, she began to self-harm by cutting and she developed an alcohol dependence to reduce her anxiety. The feeling that others could read her mind, and her critical voices caused her a lot of anxiety. She had her first admission to hospital. When she was discharged, she stopped work, and this was when her partner stopped work to look after her, and this continued for a decade or more. She had had several admissions to psychiatric hospitals and recently had been discharged after an admission to help her withdraw from benzodiazepines. She had been prescribed Valium and had been taking very high doses for years.

First Phase of the Therapy

At the beginning of the therapy, the sessions were filled with her recounting the various problems that had occurred since I last saw her. I saw her once a fortnight, in the evening. We worked on strategies to deal with her anxiety and her mood. These included keeping a diary of her mood, using relaxation exercises and mindfulness meditation. Trying to improve her mood was the main focus at the beginning. One strategy was behavioural activation. This proved quite difficult as she had a longstanding dislike of organised activities. She found going to any structured activity draining. She did have a number of acquaintances whom she enjoyed spending time with, and she was already doing this. I addressed her strategies for coping during a crisis and she had a number of different activities which she would undertake to self-soothe. She would retreat to her room and watch old TV series and listen to music. Her day-night cycle had become disturbed and she would sleep early and wake in the early hours of the morning. She had got used to living in this way for many years. I asked her about friendships and she explained that she found it easy to get on with people when she met them, but letting them close was a different thing and she had no close confiding relationships. The diary of her mood involved, in the standard way, rating her mood on a 7-point scale and keeping a note of what was going on at the time when her mood worsened, or was particularly good. This was very informative. From this, it became clear that a lot of her deteriorating mood was related to rumination about her life problems, her mother, or her financial difficulties. It also became clear that she had difficulty with any new task. She seemed to find it difficult to take in new information. But it wasn't clear whether or not this problem was due to her anxiety clouding her mind. For example, later, once she had regained her driving licence, she would only get fuel from petrol stations which didn't have a "pay at the pump" option. She thought that the "pay at the pump" option was compulsory and she was too embarrassed to go into the shop to ask for help. Feeling unable to cope with practical challenges of life was a recurring theme. When her girlfriend had been around she had sorted out most of the practical problems.

One feature of the therapy was that I was idealised from the beginning. She complained about how she was treated by the psychiatrist (and she could be quite sarcastic about her psychiatrist). He was compared negatively to me. She had reason to feel let down by her family and she regarded almost all her family very negatively. She enjoyed superficial contact with people but, as I came to know her, I began to see that under the surface she regarded people with distrust and fear. These feelings about people really emerged when she got close to them. However, this was not how she appeared on a superficial level, and most of the people she met obviously liked her. Many of her carers ended up as her friends.

Second Phase of the Therapy

Once the immediate crisis that had brought her into therapy had passed, I considered working on her delusion or on her voices. Sandra's delusions about being a Martian and people being able to read her mind did not come up as problems in what she brought to therapy. She brought relevant life problems along and she talked about her low mood, but the delusions did not feature in these discussions. It seemed counter-productive to bring them into therapy when they were not bothering her. Sometimes the voices and visions distressed her, but mainly what bothered her was far more prosaic— being depressed and thinking about killing herself, worrying about where she will live, and coping with her physical disability and chronic pain. From a cognitive therapy perspective, it would not make sense to work on delusions that are not generating distress (Chadwick, 2006; Nelson, 2005). She did, however, sometimes report distress due her voices. Sometimes when she was feeling suicidal, it would be the voices which were goading her or telling her to kill herself, so this gave a reason to work on them.

We worked on the voices using voice-dialogue. Paul Chadwick (2006) suggests this type of approach as do Byrne and colleagues (Byrne et al., 2006). Byrne and colleagues note that the person's relationship to their voices is an interpersonal relationship in which the person often feels there is a power imbalance. They argue that this need not have been how people relate to voices. The hallucination is personified and often the person will believe that the voices are a person or person-like being trying to control them. (I reproduce a transcript of a session of voice dialogue later.)

Psychodynamic Formulation

A psychodynamic model of Sandra's problems frames her psychotic symptoms as related to her other problems in life, as a sign of regression to a more primitive mental state and as being associated with impairment in relationship to other people. There are a couple of points about Sandra that are worth consideration. In terms of personal relationships, she was clearly capable of making them. She had been in a relationship for 20 years (although this had mainly been unhappy). She had several friends and acquaintances whom she saw regularly. On the other hand, she kept people at a distance. She was able to handle relationships that did not become too intense. She had no close friends. Her relationships with her family were all negative and she found herself living back near, and having daily contact with, her mother whom she said was critical and uncaring. She had a good relationship with her GP whom she saw weekly. She valued her psychotherapy sessions and attended consistently. The psychodynamic emphasis on the transference is a helpful here. It is difficult to look at Sandra's story without seeing the psychotic symptoms as part of her other difficulties and her traumatic childhood. The analytic model sees the clients account of their past as likely a distortion based on their current state of mind. It seems probable that this is true. Of course, it doesn't seem very likely that the client's past is a complete fabrication, and it is unhelpful to think that it is, in that the client will feel invalidated by this perspective. But it's unlikely that anyone's account of their childhood is an unbiased narrative, of course (Bartlett, 1932).

Her psychotic symptoms can be thought of in the following way. The hallucinated voices tell her to kill herself or cut herself. These voices are her thoughts and impulses projected into the environment, into disembodied beings of some type. She herself had no idea what to make of the voices, only that she didn't doubt that they were external voices. (There is some confusion in the psychiatric and psychological literature about this notion of "external". The expression "inner" can mean inside something, e.g. a box or a head or it can mean subjective, as in in my image of a stick. The image of a stick can't be located in spatial terms at all. So, when a client says that the voice is "external", it is important to clarify this. For example, if it's in space it can be pointed to.) Sandra never thought that the voices were her own thoughts. Her voices were heard as some being telling her to harm herself—"Kill Yourself". This is in the second person and directed to her, which implies it is from someone else. This is an example of psychotic splitting and projection. One part of her mind (an inner abusive parent) attacks another part of her mind (inner victimised child). (This, of course, happens in people who are not psychotic. But in this case, the client is not aware of this and takes the inner parent for an external being of some type, which is what makes it psychotic.)

Although Sandra said that her parents, in particular her mother, were harsh and critical, and she was neglected, and sexually abused, no one actually told her to cut herself or to kill herself. Thus, the inner critical voice is harsher than the harsh models on which it is based. This hallucinated voice demonstrates a split in the Self where one part of the mind acts as a separate self and relates to the client as someone else. Sandra also had visual hallucinations. These were always of her dead father. In these hallucinations, she felt that he was not dead, although she also knew that he was. Her late father would be looking at her in a malevolent way, although she was not sure why. This can be explained in the same way as the voices. The vision is a part of her inner world. Here she continues to be in a relationship with her dead father and in the vision, he is critical and uncaring. It is the same relationship. She also believed that she was a Martian. She thought that she had been born on Mars, was not the biological daughter of her parents and was of a different race to the rest of mankind. This seems to be an unconscious symbolic expression of her feelings of alienation and of being an outsider. It is a type of concrete thinking. Because she asserts this as true this is a delusional belief. If she said that she felt "as if" she was a Martian we would have no trouble understanding her. We can understand her belief that the voices and visions are external to her and that she is a Martian as resulting from a change in her thinking to "primary process thinking". That is the sort of thinking that Freud thought was present in dream thinking, which is not governed by the rules of logic. The idea that she is a Martian is an example of concrete thinking. Due to childhood trauma, she withdraws from people and regresses psychologically. She projects out feelings of hostility into the environment and begins to relate to figures of her imagination rather than people in the real world.

Sometimes she experienced other people reading her mind. This can be understood as the breakdown of the barriers of the self so that one begins to feel that other people have access to ones thoughts. The distinction between me and other people begins to break down. She then felt persecuted by other people who could read her mind, so that there is no barrier between her and others. Thought of in these terms, this is a very strange, deep change in how the world is experienced.

In Sandra's case, this process did not dominate most of her life. She did not spend most of her time relating to these hallucinated figures. But she did retreat from other people. She avoided close relationships with others. If she had known someone for more than a short period of time, she would become wary of them. In addition to her psychotic symptoms, we can also understand some of her other difficulties in this way. She thought of most people with a degree of suspicion. She felt controlled by her mother, as if she was a teenager again. She felt her family were trying to leave her with the minimum amount of money and that they were going to make her homeless. These ideas certainly were not psychotic, and they had basis in reality, but they also had a similar theme to her delusional belief. When a niece wanted to visit her, she did all she could to avoid it even though she had no reason to distrust her niece, and in some ways felt sympathetic to her. She had set up a pattern of avoidance that prevented her from discovering that some people could be trusted.

Sandra's idealisation of me is a way of establishing a relationship, and she valued coming along. She found the opportunity to be able to tell someone about what had been happening in her life helpful. Here, like a lot of other clients with psychosis, she was in the position of having no other close confiding relationships. This puts a lot of emphasis on the relationship with the therapist. But the relationship remained thin in that she excluded negative feelings about me. One way in which I worked with her was to draw attention to possible negative feelings towards me. For example, one session was being conducted on Zoom. She had been talking about how various things had been going wrong for her. Her brother had visited her and told her that her mother was going to have to sell the house. She didn't have enough income to rent so this was a significant threat—she might be left homeless. Also, her dog had been injured and although it wasn't a serious injury, she felt overwhelmed by having to take the dog to the vet, and she was worried about the cost. Furthermore, her health problems had been worse and she had been in pain. She felt overwhelmed. This was a typical session. She was relying on me, not so much to solve the problems, which I don't think she thought I could do, but to hear them. Alternatively, it could be that, in imagination, she felt that if she could tell me about the problems, she could leave them with me when she left. The internet connection was quite slow, and at first, we had some delay, but later we began to get freezing of the image, so that she saw me frozen on a couple of occasions.

"Simon, are you still there? Has it frozen? Or have you gone to sleep?"

I think that for her the idea that I might have fallen asleep on her seemed possible and terrifying. Her fear was of being with someone who was supporting her who then changed from a good person to a bad and unreliable person. I think that she also feared that she was too much for others and just as she had felt overwhelmed by events in her life, I now had been overwhelmed by her and I had disappeared, gone to sleep. Or, possibly, underneath that feeling, the belief that she might have metaphorically killed me off. Now there would be little point saying most of this to her, particularly with regard to her hostile feelings towards me, as she wouldn't see the link between the screen freezing and her feeling that she hated me. I suggested that in that moment when the screen froze, she feared that I had turned from a caring and listening therapist into a therapist that found her boring and didn't care about her. She didn't acknowledge that this was true but she didn't reject it either. Another example turned on the ending of the sessions. After a few years of once-a-week therapy she began to become anxious around the end of the sessions. As the session was ending, she began to ask if she had done anything wrong. This began to happen at the end of each session. I suggested that when the session ended, she asked me this because she felt that I was ending the session because I was angry with her and that she was being punished. She agreed with this, so I linked this reaction (a therapist–client link) to her feelings about her mother (a therapist—past link). She thought this made sense. She also became very aware of me looking at my watch towards the end of the sessions and she would try to catch me out looking at my watch to see if we were near the end of the session. This became something of a game, and she really was quite good at noticing me glancing at my watch.

She often compared me favourably to her psychiatrist or to other care workers, telling me how rubbish they were. I would talk about the defensive function of these comments. For example, I would suggest that it felt very important to make sure that I didn't think that she had any negative feelings about me as I might get angry and retaliate. This is important because it would be unhelpful to go along with the idea that I was some perfect therapist and that the other carers were all incompetent or malicious.

Implications for Cognitive Therapy of Psychosis

Talking about links between psychotic symptoms and other life problems is only likely to be helpful if this will make sense to the client. Usually, it won't. In Sandra's case, the positive psychotic symptoms were not her most pressing problem; however, seeing her symptoms from a psychodynamic perspective puts her relationships with people, both past and present, at the centre of her problems. Working on her relationships to others (including the therapist) is working on her psychotic problem, seen in this interpersonal way. The primary way this was evident was her anxious attachment to me and wanting to keep everything peaceful between us.

Counter-transference

Another useful aspect of this formulation is to help the therapist to be aware of his or her reaction to the client. At one point in the therapy, I started to find it difficult to follow what Sandra was saying and then I became inattentive and drowsy, and at one point she noticed this. (This was a different occasion to the one mentioned earlier, but it is obviously related to it and puts the previous example in a different light. Probably her perception wasn't completely off the mark.) I tried to understand my reaction. Usually there were a number of difficulties in her life, but these were often not interpersonal difficulties. She might be beset by a general low mood, or she might be in pain and having a series of doctors' appointments; these were quite repetitive, but this didn't really explain my reaction. I began to think about it as a reflection of her problems in some way. One possibility is that this was a repetition. She had told me that as a child she had been neglected and abused. Now in the counter-transference, she had a therapist who was losing concentration when she spoke to him. In a situation like this, it is, of course, unhelpful, particularly with a psychotic client, to suggest that my inattentiveness is something that they are bringing along although, following the model, it might be. The reason that this would be unhelpful is that the client is likely to feel blamed or that they have a therapist who won't take responsibility for his own actions. What was helpful was to not blame myself for this either, but to accept it as part of the developing process of our relationship. On reflection I realised that a lot of the material that she brought was in the nature of a complaint. I was the audience to an unremitting series of complaints; not about me but about the world, where there were no solutions and just a long future of trying to cope and there was something about this that was quite dead or deadening.

At one point, the services which usually came around and took her out were unable to come for a period of some months due to staffing difficulties. Sandra spent a lot of time alone at home and her voices became more of a problem to her. In addition to exploring coping strategies to deal with the voices, I also used a dialogue with her voices, using an empty chair as a physical representation of the disembodied voice (Perls et al., 1951; Young et al., 2003; Young & Lindemann, 1992). This technique obviously originates in the ideas of a split in the self from psychoanalysis, but it was developed as a technique by Fritz Perls (Perls et al., 1951) and is characteristic of Gestalt therapy. It has also been adopted in Schema-Focused therapy (Young et al., 2003).

Transcripts of Sessions

I will now present some transcripts of sessions with Sandra.

Voice Dialogue

Therapist:	Have the voices been a problem for you this week?
Client:	This week?
Therapist:	Yeah, or when, when was the last time they were a problem for you? When did they bother you last?
Client:	I can't remember which week.
Therapist:	Can you remember the incident?
Client:	Yes. I was down.
Therapist:	You were feeling down. And where were you?
Client:	I was at home.
Therapist:	And what were the voices saying?
Client:	They kept saying "They will kill you; They will kill you; they'll kill you"
Therapist:	"They are going to kill you". And what did the voices mean by that?
Client:	The voices meant me.
Therapist:	Who was the "they" that was going to kill you? So, were they saying "We're going to kill you" is that what they said?
Client:	No, no, the voices were going over and over. "They are going to kill you; they are going to kill you"
Therapist:	Who did they mean? Do you know?
Client:	I'm not sure I'm not sure.
Therapist:	And what do you make of the voices? What do you think they are?
Client:	It's all different, it's all different. Um. (pause) It's not always the same, you know?
Therapist:	Yeah.
Client:	Sometimes its alien voices, sometimes other people's voices, sometimes it's like several different voices like all in a crowd, you know?
Therapist:	If we pick one of them causes you the most trouble, do you know which one it would be? Would be the aliens or . . . ?
Client:	Um . . . (To herself) What would be the worst? I mean my father . . .
Therapist:	. . . That's bad?
Client:	yeah that's disturbing.
Therapist:	All right let's imagine your father's voice, that is the voice that you hear of your father, not when he was

	alive, but the voice you hear now, is in the chair (pointing to an empty chair) okay? And then we can have a bit of a conversation with the voice to see where we go, okay, how would that be?
Client:	Right. But how could it be . . . not when he was alive, how can I think of him? When he was dead? (laughs) You know like . . .
Therapist:	You don't think of him as dead, though, do you?
Client:	I'm not sure he is dead but he comes back (laughs)
Therapist:	Maybe just think of him as the voice that you hear that bothers you. So, it doesn't have to be alive or dead just that voice. When it bothers you.
Client:	Right.
Therapist:	Whether he's alive or dead doesn't matter. For these purposes it doesn't matter.
Client:	Right. Okay, okay.
Client (softly):	"Mad bitch"
Therapist:	Right. Well now the voice is over there (indicating the chair) I'm not going to get you to jump between chairs because of your leg. But he is saying "Mad bitch". What else does he say?
Client:	(louder). "Mad bitch. No other parents would put up with you!"
Therapist:	He still says that to you, does he? So mad bitch. No one else would ever want you.
Client:	Yes. "You're useless. Not good at anything. No one in the family can stand you"
Therapist:	Right. Ok. Yeah (pause) so pretty horrible, huh? And did he talk that way when he was alive? To you?
Client:	Yes oh yes.
Therapist:	So hearing the voice is a bit like him being . . .
Client:	. . . It's a bit like a recording of when he was alive.
Therapist:	So "Mad bitch no one likes you"
Client:	Yes. "No-one in the family likes you"
Therapist:	You're useless?
Client:	Yes.
Therapist:	Okay so imagine he's over there. What would you want to say to the voice?
Client:	Umm . . . I'm torn between telling him off (laughs)
Therapist:	Yeah.
Client:	. . . and feeling that he's right about everything.
Therapist:	What's he doing it for? Why is he saying those things to you?
Client:	Why is he saying them? He's punishing me . . .
Therapist:	Punishing you? Well maybe that isn't very good should we try to talk to him about that?

Client:	Umm.
Therapist:	What would you like to say to him?
Client. (Pause):	That's a good question. (Pause). He wouldn't answer.
Therapist:	What can we say? What would you say to him?
Client:	Why do you always want to punish me?
Therapist:	Yes, that's a good one. Why do you always want to punish me? And what do you think about him punishing you? What do you think of it?
Client:	It worries me because I try and go over and over in my head what I'd done → that's so bad. You know and then I try to fight thinking . . .
Therapist:	You think you have done something bad enough that he should want to be bad to you and punish you like that?
Client:	errrr . . . (pause) well sometimes I do and sometimes I don't (laughs)
Therapist:	Yes, you think different things at different times.
Client:	Yes.
Therapist:	What do you think about him calling you those names and stuff?
Client:	I don't know. It makes me feel down.
Therapist:	So, the part of you that wants to stand up to him what would you say, to the voice?
Client:	If I stood up to him?
Therapist:	Yeah, the part of you that wants . . . there are two parts to you. One part of you thinks that you deserve to be punished but the other bit that's feeling like you don't deserve it. What does that part want to say to the voice?
Client:	Umm. . . . Err. (Pause). Of course, I'm a mad bitch I had you as a father, didn't I?
Therapist:	(Laughs)
Client:	Actually, I can remember saying that to him. (Laughs). I did. I said of course I'm a mad bitch I had you for father, didn't I?
Therapist and Client:	(laugh)
Therapist:	I like that. How did it feel to say that to him?
Client:	(laughing) Good. And remember I did actually say to him.
Therapist:	And you did actually say it. Yes, that's very good. And how would he react to that?
Client:	(Pause). I'm blank on that one I don't know how it would respond.
Therapist:	You don't know how he would respond?
Client:	No.
Therapist:	And is there anything else you would want to say to him?

Client:	I can't think.
Therapist:	Well, suppose you said something like (talking to the empty chair) "Look it's got to stop this abuse. It's really unhelpful and when you say these things you are just trying to hurt Sandra here and really you have got to cut it out. We don't want to know about that thank you very much. It's not helpful". How would that feel to say that to him?
Client:	It's hard because I now realise it was abuse. You know . . .
Therapist:	What do you think? Am I right? Is it abuse?
Client:	I know now its abuse but I always thought that to be abuse you had to be beat up.
Therapist:	Yes you always thought being abused meant being hit.
Client:	Yes, I never thought of other things . . . yeah . . . being abused. It's only now I know. Abuse is all sorts of things, isn't it?
Therapist:	Of course . . . Calling someone a mad bitch is a bit abusive.
Client:	Yes, verbal abuse; sexual abuse; What's the other one?
Therapist:	Emotional?
Client:	Emotional. Emotional.
Therapist:	So, if you say to the voice, I'm a mad bitch I had you as a father. Or cut it out. Stop it! How do you think the voice will respond?
Client:	(Pause). How will he respond to that? I'm not sure.
Therapist:	How does it feel now talking to the voice like that?
Client:	Umm. I don't know.
Therapist:	Is it good or bad or neutral?
Client:	Yes neutral. Maybe more good than bad, I think. Yeah. More good than bad.
Therapist:	Is there a bad feeling about doing it?
Client:	No. Just a bit funny talking to the chair (laughs)
Therapist:	(Laughs). Yes, talking to a chair (laughs) Yes that's right.
Therapist:	It is funny talking to a chair, isn't it? But. I'm doing it as well.
Client:	(laughs)
Therapist:	We are both talking to a chair (pause) So, if we say to the voice "Why are you doing this? Why are you punishing Sandra like this? What was the point?" If we said "Why would you want to be spending your time, making Sandra feel bad" what would it say?
Client:	(pause)

Therapist:	Well, what do you think the reason for it is? Why would it want to do that, spend its time trying to put you down?
Client:	(pause). Punish me. It was the same with my girlfriend.
Therapist:	Your girlfriend treated you the same?
Client:	Yes. She would always be calling me names or criticising me.
Therapist:	What for?
Client:	For doing things wrong.
Therapist:	What have you done wrong?
Client:	Not being able to do things that other people do.
Therapist:	What like?
Client:	Talking to people.
Therapist:	She didn't like you talking to people?
Client:	Oh yeah, she used to get cranky if I talked to other people.
Therapist:	. . . Really?
Client:	Oh yeah, she didn't like if I talked to other people. I talked people over the fence and she embarrassed me she said "Come on you've been talking too long": I said "Why?" and she said "You've been talking enough"
Therapist:	So, she wouldn't let you talk to people?
Client:	She was jealous I know that.
Therapist:	Why else might she be doing it?
Client:	To punish me.
Therapist:	To punish you because you couldn't do things is that what you mean?
Client:	Yeah. I didn't do anything right; you know what I mean? I was never allowed in the kitchen. You know.
Therapist:	She wouldn't let you go in the kitchen?
Client:	No.
Therapist:	Because she didn't like how you cooked?
Client:	Because I didn't put the cups the right way.
Therapist:	She sounds a bit controlling, from what you say.
Client:	Yes, I know that now that she was controlling.
Therapist:	So, do you think the voice is trying to control you.
Client:	Yes. Yes.
Therapist:	So, it's about punishment but the motive of the voice is to control you?
Client:	Yes, I didn't realise that until now but everything she did was controlling. What I wear.
Therapist:	Was that what she was like?
Client:	Oh yeah. If I was getting myself dressed up it would be like, where are you going? I don't want you going down the shop with make up on.

Therapist: Do you think it might be, I mean I don't know, but, that she was worried that she might lose you if she didn't keep you under control? If you are allowed to just be a person, go around and do your stuff maybe you would realise that there were some better options or something like that? Do you think?

Client: There probably were some better options.

Therapist: I mean I wonder if she was insecure?

Client: Yeah, I know you mean. But I mean . . . it's me . . . (Laughs) how could anybody be interested . . . in me? (Laughs) I forgot that word.

Therapist: Insecure.

Client: Yeah. Maybe she was scared that I would tell her I wanted to leave home.

Therapist: Yeah, maybe she was scared you'd meet somebody else and leave.

Client: Yeah. But in the end, I did.

Commentary

In this role play, there are two levels to this interaction. At one level, we are obviously role playing an interaction with her voices. The role play is an attempt to help her to change her relationship with the voice. This is related to Byrne and colleagues' (2006) work on changing the interpersonal relationship to the voices or Chadwick's (2006) work on confronting the voices using the two-chair technique to the same end. It is a technique from Gestalt Therapy (Perls et al., 1951) used in Schema therapy to try to change the client's relationship with parts of the self. As this dialogue develops, the client moves from a conversation with a critical and punitive voice to a dialogue with her late-father, and then to a dialogue with her ex-partner. Sandra isn't clear that her father is dead. In one way, she knows that he is and, in another way, she doesn't think he is. This is a puzzling state of mind. What are we to make of it? I think this is an example of the less obvious type of psychotic symptom. The boundary between what is real and what is not and the boundary between the living and the dead have become blurred. She is confused about whether this is a dialogue with her late-father or a part of her mind. Also, she is unsure if the dead are dead or whether they might be dead and not-dead at the same time. Freud says that a characteristic of primary process thinking is that logic is ignored and associations are determined by affective links. This type of symptom is mentioned less in DSM and ICD-10 possibly because it is harder to operationalise.

I am trying to encourage her to stand up to the voice by coaching and cheerleading her to be more assertive towards the voice. Incidentally, an alternative approach is to be less directive about this and allow the dialogue with the voice in the chair to develop. As well as encouraging the client to be more assertive with a controlling part of the self, another outcome can be an increase in understanding of the other person. This might have been the case, for example, when Sandra was talking to her ex-girlfriend. It is less true when dealing with a voice which is not so much a person but more a persecutory part-object. That is a voice that is more purely bad or evil, in so far as the voice turns out to be purely motivated by malice or hatred.

The second level of this role play is her relationship to me in therapy. With this perspective, she is cooperating in a role play that I suggest will help her. The role play is about standing up to a critical voice. But in the session, she is going along with my suggestion that this role play will help her. This may encourage the feeling that the therapist is an ideal person who has some magical power to fix her problems; that is, it may encourage an idealisation of the therapist. The problem with this, of course, is not only that it is unreal but also that idealisation goes hand in hand with denigration, being idealised switches easily into being denigrated. Or if the therapist is idealised, then often the other people in the client's life are denigrated.

She doubted her abilities to navigate the world. Her ex-partner was much older than her and she had a psychotic breakdown and gave up work soon after meeting her. Her partner then gave up work and became her carer. So, this was her relationship, Sandra in the role of sick and incapable and her partner in the role of caring for her. After they separated, she was free of an external persecutor, but at the same time she felt left alone in a world where she couldn't function. She had no confidence in her ability to solve simple practical problems (e.g. on one occasion, she sat in darkness as she doubted her ability to following instructions about resetting a circuit breaker). This reflects a sense of the world as hostile and her as weak and vulnerable.

These reflections are useful in the following way. It is important not to buy into the idea of Sandra as weak and therapist as strong and good, because this merely confirms the ongoing system. By buying into the idea of the therapist as strong, this implicitly reinforces the idea that the client cannot do it on her own.

Session Transcript

The client had confirmed her appointment the previous day. As it was raining heavily, she sent an SMS saying that she would prefer to Skype rather than come in. In the previous session, I had altered her regular appointment time to the mid-afternoon from midday. This had meant that she couldn't come in and we had had to meet on Skype the previous week.

Client:	Hello Simon. (pause) I feel terrible.
Therapist:	Why? What's going on?
Client:	I feel terrible. I'm sorry I have been stuffing you around.
Therapist:	How do you mean?

Client:	Well I said that I was coming yesterday and then today I messaged you to say I couldn't come in due to the rain. I got up and I was going to come but the rain was heavy. It was running down the side of the house and then back towards this ridge on the window. That's when I know that it's really heavy. I felt terrible about not coming in. I would hate for you to be annoyed.
Therapist:	So you feel that you may be talking to a therapist who feels annoyed that you didn't get in and that you should have been trying harder?
Client:	Yes that it! Only when you say it, it sounds odd.
Therapist:	Well I think that it sounds odd because there is a part of you that expects me to be thinking to myself "How dare she rearrange the appointment because of a little rain?" and another part of you that doubts that.
Client:	I'd hate for you to be pissed off with me.
Therapist:	You hate it when people change your appointments and you hated it when I changed your appointment last week and you feel that I might feel that too.
Client:	It was because it was the idea that someone else was in my appointment time that I didn't like it.
Therapist:	Yes.

A little later, she continued

Client:	The bookkeeper had said that he wasn't doing my brother's tax for him this year. My brother's wife is a bookkeeper I told him. So, he said "Well why doesn't she do his tax for him?" (pause) A strange thing happened, I was on the computer, and an ad on something I had been talking about flashed up on the screen.
Therapist:	What did you make of that?
Client:	It seemed weird like the computer knew what I had been talking about. It made me think about cameras in the house again. I have been feeling overloaded. It's been a difficult week. I have been hearing this mumbling all the time.
Therapist:	Mumbling?
Client:	Yes. I hear these voices but they are talking on top of each other so I can't tell what they are saying but it's been going on all the time. Like voices at a rock concert all mixed up.
Therapist:	What do you make of it?
Client:	What do I make of it?
Therapist:	Yes. Do you feel it's your imagination or that it's coming from outside?

Client:	It's not my imagination. It's coming from my head. It sounds like it's coming from inside my head and then going outside from my head.
Therapist:	Do you think other people can hear it?
Client:	No. They can't. I was here yesterday seeing Dr _ and when I was in the waiting room, I was watching people and they didn't pay any attention. They just carried on with their mobile phones or whatever and didn't pay any attention at all.
Therapist:	You mean you watched people and as they didn't react, they can't be hearing it?
Client:	Yes.
Therapist:	Why do you think others can't hear them?
Client:	I don't know. I saw Dr _ yesterday and I watched him and he didn't react.
Therapist:	What do you make of these voices?
Client:	I don't know. They are one of the world's mysteries.
Therapist:	Well there are a few of those aren't there?
Client:	Yes.
Therapist:	And how have you been feeling?
Client:	I have been feeling down and depressed for a while.
Therapist:	When did the mumbling start?
Client:	Well it must have, let's see, today is Friday, it was there on Wednesday and . . . I think it started last weekend.
Therapist:	And what was going on at that time?
Client:	Nothing really. Well, my bookkeeper came around on Thursday. There had been some problems with Jane arguing about the money.
Therapist:	So you feel that he is on your side?
Client:	He was saying that I could move out into a retirement village. I was a bit worried about that. He said it's not a nursing home. It's for over 55's and I would have my own rooms and a court-yard. He said that I wouldn't have to worry about Jane anymore then.
Therapist:	So he was being helpful, but with your family and Jane and the others, you feel sometimes that no one is on your side.
Client:	This week I have been so impatient. When people come around, I just want them to go. Even my support worker Susan. She called up and asked if I wanted to go for coffee and I said that I was just going to bed. I wasn't as it was only 3:30 (pm) but I didn't want to see her.
Therapist:	Maybe the feeling irritated and the mumbling are related to the feeling that your ex is prepared to sell you down the river.
Client:	Hmm. I just don't want people around.
Therapist:	Wanting to push people away does that apply here with me?

Client:	No not here. It's different here. I get listened to here.
Therapist:	So it doesn't feel the same as with friends.
Client:	I have been tearing up photos. I went through all my photos and all of the photos with my brother. I tore them up and his children. I kept some of Jane and me and the cats.
Therapist:	It was a satisfying feeling.
Client:	. . . getting back at them.
	. . . My mother got a good result with her cancer. They operated and they got it all. Also, I have lost 15 kg. Since I was diagnosed as having diabetes, I need to lose weight.
Therapist:	That's good! When you diet are you ever tempted to lose too much again?
Client:	No. My mother was bulimic you know. She still watches her calories and she now weighs 42 kg.

Commentary

This session is unusual in that Sandra brings along her voices. The session opens with Sandra's anxiety about our relationship. She has changed the medium of the therapy from face to face to video link. She is obviously very concerned that she will have upset me by changing her mind on the day. However, the previous week I had changed the appointment time from noon to the afternoon and this had entailed having to carry out the session by video link rather than face to face. So it may be that her concerns about her changing the appointment also reflect a protest against me for having cancelled her session the previous week. She has been hearing the mumbling for over a week. It sounds like many voices talking over each other. She can't hear what they are saying but she has the sense that they are malevolent. She doesn't think that the voices are in her mind. She doesn't think that they are imaginary and she has to deduce that other people can't hear them from the reactions of other people. No one is looking to see where the voices are from. So, her experience of these voices is that they are perceptions rather than thoughts. Also, she cannot make out what they say. This doesn't fit the phenomenology of thoughts at all. Furthermore, she has the sense that the voices are emanating from inside her head and are travelling outwards. And she is *surprised* that others cannot hear them. When I try to clarify her understanding of the voices, she says that she doesn't know what they are. She doesn't have a delusional elaboration of these experiences (on this occasion). It would be possible to work cognitively on these voices by setting up a rival hypothesis, or to work on changing her relationship to the voices. What I attempt do to instead is to clarify when and where the voices began. I am trying to contextualise the voices and to see if it is possible to link them to other aspects of her life. The voices have been around at the same time that she has had a number of problems in her life, For example, one life problem is her bookkeeper confirming her fears about Sandra's partner and family. This is the experience of her life. Her response to this is to cut the photographs of all the people in her family who she hated. In the previous role play, the client and the therapist role play expressing feelings towards her voices/father/girl-friend. In the present case, there is nothing of the role play about it at all. Sandra expresses her feelings towards her brother and her mother by symbolically destroying them. She shares this experience with the therapist who witnesses this and this involves her becoming closer to the therapist by sharing these feelings. It seems that by listening to the client and clarifying her feelings a similar end is reached as by getting her to act it out. Only the second example is surely preferable as it was Sandra's idea to cut up the photographs and to share this with me. And I become a "good object" in the transference.

The psychotic symptom here seems to be part of an emotional reaction to a specific situation. The client was worried about the security of her housing, but more importantly she feels that she is being treated by her ex-partner and her family as if her needs do not matter. She does not assert herself or express her anger about this situation. This situation reminds her of many previous situations. Being shouted at and criticised, being hit, being called crazy, being abused. The mumbling voices are the background to this. They are an expression of her feelings, which present themselves to her as perceptions rather than emotions. Mainly here I am trying to link her feelings to the events that have been going on. The timing of the events doesn't always fit with this, but I develop a theory with her as the session develops, which is that she feels devastated and let down and that the mumbling is a part of this.

The session opens with her anxieties about having let me down, and I talk to her about her perception of me as an unreasonable critic (which she half acknowledges). I make some reference to the previous session in which we were on video link because I had changed the time of the session from her usual slot to the middle of the afternoon. She thinks I have done this to accommodate another client so the accusation about being never put first can be applied to me in this case, and she is able to acknowledge this which is, of course, very helpful.

As Sandra rarely presents delusional ideas in the session, I don't focus on them. But the idea that she is a Martian and being told to kill herself and that she is useless by the voices both fit in with her idea of herself as worthless. And this relates to her experience of abuse. Why do people who are abused as children often have low self-esteem? One possibility is that if the person has been victimised over a period of time, they have internalised an Abuser—Victim role pair and that they enact this towards themselves where one part of them is identified with the abuser and the other part with the victim.

The session can be read as having a paranoid theme. Her brothers are confirmed as "terrible people" and her financial advisor (who she has had serious doubts about in the past, thinking that he was exploiting her or acting for her brothers) now is seen as a hero figure. So, there is a splitting of the "object" into a good and bad (good and bad breast to use the Kleinian language. The point of the "breast" as opposed to "person" here is that the "object" is not a person (with a variety of good and bad traits) but a part-object, with wholly good or bad traits. The bad traits have been projected out into the part-object).

I think that one of the things she found particularly painful was not knowing whether she could trust her instincts about people. She doubted her ability to judge. Sometimes it is safer to assume that people are bad if you aren't sure rather than to risk being wrong.

An important part of the session was when Sandra agreed that she had not liked having her appointments changed and that this had annoyed her. She didn't agree to negative feelings about me very much, usually saying that her idealised view of me was how it actually was rather than the way she like to see things.

A Later Session

Due to physical problems, primarily pain, I had seen her on video call on a number of occasions. This had worked quite well. She began by apologising for not coming into the practice. She said that she felt that she was letting everyone down recently. She had come in to see the doctor yesterday not only because she needed to get the results of her recent tests but also because she wanted to find out the cause of the shooting pain she had developed in her arms and legs. Could it be, she wondered, a reaction to a new medication she had been given? She had been given the medication about 10 days before the pains began. The doctor had thought not but said that he couldn't be 100% sure about this. She had cancelled her workers from various NGO's who were to come around and help her out. One worker had taken her dog to the vet and the dog had been given worming tablets but these tablets had been the wrong tablets and her dog had started to vomit. I commented that when this sort of crisis happened, she couldn't exactly take the dog to the vet herself and she had few people that she could rely on to back her up. She said she had no one apart from various workers. She worries about what would happen to her if she were admitted to hospital. When she goes into hospital and they ask her for her next of kin she doesn't know who to put. She could put her mother but that isn't what they want, they want someone who could be called if there was a problem or something and her mother being confined to a nursing home wasn't really what they needed. And there wasn't anyone. I said that she never thought of asking one of her brothers to come down and look after her dog. She said that she didn't ever think of that and that she was really on her own.

Commentary

In this session, there is a theme of her being alone in an uncaring world. There is someone who is supposed to help who inflicts damage instead. Her doctor gives her a medicine that she thinks may have caused the pain; the vet gives her dog a medicine which makes the dog vomit. And if she is in hospital, there is no one to look after her dog or her affairs. Her ex-partner and her family want to cheat her out of her savings.

Sandra's delusional beliefs are that she comes from Mars and that other people can read her mind. Her sense of isolation is expressed by her belief in being a Martian and her current feelings about not being thought about by her mother. She felt that her family were currently actively conspiring against her, to evict her from her home and leave her with as little as possible. This can be thought of as a projection of her inner rejecting parent onto her brothers and her elderly, institutionalised, and dependant mother, but I thought that there was a good deal of truth about her feelings. For example, her bookkeeper had warned her that her ex-partner was trying to take her to the cleaners financially.

Sandra's idea that other people could read her mind is clearly a standard psychotic experience. What should we make of this? It is an example of the breakdown of the boundaries of the self. But the boundaries of the Self do not break down in a neutral way. The breakdown allows thoughts of inadequacy to surface and her personal identity is violated.

A Later Session

In a later session, Sandra began by talking about her physical problems and her chronic pain. Due to her knee problem, she has limped for many years. And this has now led to problems with her back. She has recently been getting a feeling like lightning going down her legs. This is probably some arthritic condition and this has led to her being stuck in the house which leads to being depressed and having thoughts about sticking a knife in the toaster. She had been feeling in pain and had been about to go bed (at 2 pm) and then the post had arrived. When she got the post, it was an official letter asking her to contact her financial advisor's office as she had to sign a form and pay a bill. She had been looking forward to sleeping but now couldn't as she was anxious about the form and what it might mean. She had called her accountant, but when she got through to the office, she had been told that he was away on annual leave looking after a family member. She told the receptionist that she had him in order to deal with exactly this sort of form and claim and that she wasn't able to do it. The receptionist said that she would have to wait until her returned in a week to find out what the form was about.

After this, she said, there had been confusion from the NGO about who her support person was going to be on various days. Different people had said different things. I said that when things went wrong, she felt as if the world was always going to throw problems at her and that she wouldn't have the ability to cope with it. She agreed with this. I said that it was as if it was the same as when she was a child. She agreed with this but went on to say that there were actually no options at the moment as well. At the very end of the session, she explained that she hears voices most of the time. I asked her what she thought they were. She said that she used to be sure that they were aliens—Martians. Now she is only 80% sure. And then sometimes she hears the voice of the Devil. And she knows that it's the Devil when he speaks and he tells her to harm herself or to die.

Commentary

In this session, Sandra feels surrounded by hostile demands which she is incapable of meeting, or which she worries that she will be incapable of meeting. When I attempt to describe this to her, she agrees, but then emphasises the real nature of the current demands on her. And the problem about the payment from the accounting agency had not been resolved. She feels that the worst thing about this is that she will be unable to cope with the demands made on her. Her comments at the end of the session about continually hearing voices of aliens and less frequently the voice of the Devil seem to relate to what she has been talking about throughout the session as a response to my comment about her feeling that the reality of the world was that it was always about to let her down or attack her. The voices that trouble her and predict doom are the voices of Martians and of the Devil. In Sandra's case, this daily experience of voices does not dominate the sessions. With other clients, it is the only thing that they think and talk about. She has relationships with people in the real world. She struggles with her relationship with her mother and her brother and she had emotional investment with her care workers, her GP and with me. Thinking about her current practical problems as part of the same universe that brings Martians and the Devil helps to join these problems up as one problem. With me the problem is that she can't allow there to be problems between us. Towards the end of the session, she asked me if it was nearly time to finish and said that she was wondering if she had done anything wrong (that is, was I about to end the session because she had done something to upset me). This came up as an issue frequently, so she knew that my answer was going to be that no, nothing she had done had led to the end of the session. It is important, however, to explore the meaning of this reaction, not simply offer reassurance.

A Later Session

Sandra arrived early as usual. I was expecting her to want to do the session by video. I made her a mug of coffee. She began by talking about the weather. She then went on to say that her previous support worker (Jill) had been in touch with her by text message. The support worker had said that she missed her and her dog. As Sandra had deliberately arranged not to have this worker as she didn't find her helpful this bothered her and she said that Jill was trying to worm her way back into working with her. Jill had said that she was still not working. Sandra said that she knew this wasn't true. Sandra had said that she had another worker and Jill had said this was good. Sandra had said that they should catch up for coffee and Jill had said yes straight away. Sandra regretted this. She said that she had suggested this out of guilt but didn't really want to see her at all. I reminded her that when she had had Jill as a support worker, she had always found it a problem and that she found it difficult to say "No", because she wanted other people to approve of her and avoided conflict with others. She had enough conflict in her life and avoided any more. She said that I wasn't the first person to suggest this and that other people had said that she was too nice and that others took advantage of her. I thought that this was quite likely to be true.

She told me that she was going to go with her current support worker to visit a small town and that they had a music shop which sold guitars and ukulele. She was thinking of buying a ukulele. She said that I had said that they were easy to play. I said that there were classes where one could learn with other people. She said that she didn't like groups of people. She is good at one to one with other people. But in groups she couldn't really function. I asked her what happened she said that in a group she becomes anxious. What does she fear? She said that it has always been like this. In a group, she has to be the first one there. She doesn't want to have to make an arrival. And what she fears is that the others will plot against her to hurt her. In what way? They will plot against her to harm her. They will beat her up.

Commentary

In this session, she is being pursued by someone who used to be her support worker who she thinks wants to manipulate her to having her back. She ends up suggesting that they meet even though she doesn't want this at all. She goes on to talk about being anxious in groups of people. The theme running through these two topics is her fear of other people and her inability to stand up to them. This really has been the story of her life, from childhood through her long-term lesbian relationship.

General Commentary

In these sessions, the recurring theme is of other people being persecutory—wanting to take from her or wanting to push her into something that she doesn't want to do. I feature as the negative person on a couple of occasions, but mainly I am idealised. On those occasions, I am an uninterested therapist, or I am trying to get rid of her by ejecting her from the session, or I am putting someone else in her regular therapy slot as I don't care about her. These themes are not delusional, although they are on similar themes to some of her delusional ideas (voices or the Devil wanting to harm her—being a Martian and alone in an alien world, people reading her mind and her having no privacy even in her mind). It is useful for the therapist to have these ideas in mind in dealing with a client, as being aware of the state of the relationship between the client and the therapist affects how the therapist sees the client's responses and the therapist's own response. Most obviously here my occasional lack of presence and her perception of this as rejecting and uncaring.

References

Bartlett, F. (1932). *Remembering: A study in experimental and social psychology.* Cambridge: Cambridge University Press.

Byrne, S., Birchwood, M., Trower, P. E., & Meaden, A. (2006). *Casebook of cognitive behaviour therapy for command hallucinations: A social rank theory approach.* London and New York: Routledge.

Chadwick, P. (2006). *Person based cognitive therapy for distressing psychosis.* Chichester: Wiley.

Nelson, H. (2005). *Cognitive therapy with delusions and hallucinations.* Cheltenham: Stanley Thornes.

Perls, F., Hefferline, R., & Goodman, P. (1951). *Gestalt therapy: Excitement and growth in the human personality.* New York: Julian.

Young, J. E., Klosko, J. S., & Weishaar, M. E. (2003). *Schema therapy: A practitioners guide.* New York: Guilford Press.

Young, J. E., & Lindemann, M. D. (1992). An integrative schema-focused model of personality disorders. *Journal of Cognitive Psychotherapy: An International Quarterly, 6*(1), 11–23.

7 Jane

The Fear of Revenge—A Repetition of Abuse 1

Jane was referred to a psychology clinic in Bankstown, South Western Sydney. She was a middle-aged woman who had been chronically deluded for over 20 years. She was a thin woman who was manifestly tense almost all the time. She had a number of chronic delusions which were related to experiences of reference and she also heard voices of a threatening nature. She lived on her own in a government provided flat that was two small rooms in a low-rise block, in a built up semi-suburban area. She had one brother who lived on the other side of Sydney. She couldn't see him as she found it difficult to leave the house because of her fears. I met her in a room in the psychology clinic which was located next to the Bankstown Psychiatric Inpatient ward. The clinic had once been a thriving anxiety disorders clinic but now saw a range of clients with psychosis or personality disorders. When I saw her, I had been newly appointed to the clinic and it had only one other psychologist who worked on different days to me. The clinic was full of empty rooms. The psychology manager had left, the secretary had left, and the other psychologist was on maternity leave. There was a feeling of abandonment about the place, half a dozen empty rooms, and no reception staff. It was destined to be closed down by the Health Service and it felt like an unwanted child.

She was an engaging, warm woman to talk to and she would ask me questions and make suggestions about various things. Talking with her was definitely an interaction. The main feeling that came up in being with her was her anxiety. She complained of hearing voices. She had some insight into her psychotic experiences so that she believed that she hallucinated voices. But she didn't think that all the voices she heard were hallucinations. She thought that some of the voices were people speaking through a wall or were people standing near her. And she had a great fear of these voices. Sometimes she acted on what the voices said by responding to them as one might with a real voice. Obviously this was worrying, as her behaviour could be misunderstood by other people who might, for example, react to being asked if they had called her an abusive name. She had been housebound and living alone for over 10 years, so her insight didn't really do her much good. She spent her days mostly alone in her room unless she

DOI:10.4324/9781003168379-9

ventured out to shop. She had a case manager who visited her every month to check on how she was. The voices threatened her that she would be harmed, or insulted her calling her a child molester, or worthless. She was referred for help with her voices as there seemed no further chemical solution to her psychotic symptoms.

She was the eldest of three children from a working-class Filipino family. She grew up in a small-town north of Sydney. There wasn't a lot of money to go around. She had got on ok at school and had friends; in fact, she quite liked school. The problem had been her home life. As a child, she had been terrified of her father for as long as she could remember. Her father would often go to the pub on the way home from work. Everyone would be waiting in fear to see what state of mind he would be when he got back from the pub. If he was in a bad mood, he used to beat the children. Jane had taken to hiding under the bed when her father was due home. Her mother was unable to protect her from her father. She thought that she was as scared as everyone else. She had a good relationship with one of her sisters. So, her father was an ogre and everyone was equally afraid of him. Jane wasn't singled out for abuse. As a defence Jane developed the ability to laugh when her father hit her. Unfortunately, this was a defence that provoked her father who would hit her all the more. As soon as she was old enough, she left home and got a job working in Sydney. Things went well for her until she was in her early 20s.

She began to develop some anxiety symptoms. She began having panic attacks and to feel increasingly uncomfortable in social situations. She began to worry more. There was no obvious external trigger to these symptoms. It is possible that the precipitant was developmental and that it is the change in role to becoming fully an adult, and the conflict that resisting the identification with her father might entail (resisting the return of the bad object in Fairbairn's language). It was difficult to be clear because her account of her past was coloured by her current delusions.

She saw a psychologist to help her with her panic, and then in her mid-20s, she had a psychotic breakdown. Her account of what happened was that she had agreed to import drugs into the country but then, having second thoughts backed out at the last minute. After this she quickly slid into psychosis. She recalled being in her bedroom when she began to hear a voice threatening her. She thought this was a voice of the people who had wanted her to transport the drugs. She was hearing the voices all the time. They told her that they would rape or kill her sister. It wasn't clear how she thought these voices were getting into her room. It was difficult to determine what she had thought and felt at the time and what was her interpretation looking back, but what she now believed was that the voices she heard were the drug dealers. She had stayed in her room. In the end, she had gone to the police about this situation, and informed on the men who had asked her to transport the drugs. She believed that they had been sent to prison. She thought that they would get out of jail soon and that when they did, they would come and take revenge on her by torturing and murdering her. Her main source of evidence for this was that she would hear people telling her this as she passed them in the street. (She often thought the voices she heard were from people that she was near in the street.) Maybe, most importantly, she had a strong intuition that this was the case.

Therapy

The beginning of the therapy consisted in a long period of listening to her and clarifying what she was saying. She was happy to talk about her problems and engaged quickly. As her psychotic symptoms dominated her life, we worked on techniques to deal with her voices then went on to examine the truth of her delusions using cognitive therapy. I began with Coping Skills Enhancement, using solution-focused questions as well as making suggestions about strategies to try out. A lot of this work was really about motivating her to apply techniques to deal with her voices. Distraction and using music to relax were two of the main strategies she focused on.

As she already believed that she had psychotic symptoms and that some of the voices she heard were hallucinatory, she readily agreed when I suggested testing out if she was really in danger from the drug traffickers and if the critical and abusive voices she heard were real or part of her emotional illness. We didn't have to deal with anxieties around having a mental illness or having hallucinations, because she already believed that she had schizophrenia and was hallucinating. In other clients, the idea of being psychotic or having a mental illness needs to be addressed before it's possible to examine the truth of the delusion itself (Nelson, 2005). We looked at the validity of the evidence she had for her belief and alternative interpretations of this evidence. So, for example, one source of evidence that she was in danger was that she was being threatened by voices. We explored whether what the voices said was true. She did not have evidence that the drug smugglers had gone to prison apart from the voices, but she surmised that they had done. We looked at counter evidence. When I asked her why, if they intended to harm her, the people who she had informed on had not harmed her yet, she would say that it was because they had been in prison. I asked her why had she not been called to court? Why had the police, in fact, never contacted her again after she had made her report? If there was a court case why wouldn't her evidence against them have been important, as she was a witness to them asking her to bring in drugs? Why had the police not interviewed her in more detail at the time? Why had she not heard about the case in the papers or on the news? How had the voices spoken to her in her bedroom with no one around? This had some impact on her belief in the session but it wasn't maintained between sessions, so we moved on to setting up behavioural experiments. As she heard the voices more when she was around other people, we went out to cafes where other people would be around and, when she heard a voice, I acted as the independent observer.

She would tell me when she heard a voice and I would tell her if I had heard it too. When we were out, it was easy to tell when she had heard a voice as she oriented towards the "sound" and looked visibly disturbed. When I told her that I couldn't hear the voice she accepted this, and she never questioned whether I was telling her the truth, but it didn't really affect her belief in the reality of the voices. Maybe because she already knew that she sometimes hallucinated, it wasn't news to her that she was sometimes hallucinating. The problem was that this didn't prove that she was always hallucinating. Some authors have speculated about the quasi-mental/quasi-sensory nature of voices, but in her case, it was easy to see that she heard the voices as if they were a voice located in a point in the room.

As well as being a test of the reality of the voices, these trips out were also a type of exposure programme, as in general she avoided leaving the house unless essential. She always took a cab when she was coming to see me due to her voices and her fear of being killed by someone associated with the criminals. She saw no one regularly apart from me and her case manager who saw her only once a month. So, another major part of the therapy was that she got to talk about her worries and concerns. This is a significant change in the environment. Having someone to talk to about problems when usually there is no one else to talk to at all is clearly likely to have a great impact on someone's life.

Like many withdrawn paranoid clients, most of her interactions were with her voices or other parts of reality coloured strongly by her paranoid explanations. Here is an example—she had met a stranger in the street. She had said "Hello" to him and the man had stopped and had a conversation with her. The stranger had said something to her which Jane had interpreted as meaning that she (Jane) would soon be under threat. Jane thought that he had told her that the drug traffickers would soon be released from jail. She thought that this meant that they would come after her. She took this conversation as evidence that her delusion was true, and also acted on it by going to the house where one of the group of traffickers had lived and knocking on the door. No one answered. It would have been useful to have asked her for the detail of what the person she had met actually said, as she related it by saying what she took the man to mean. Given that I didn't believe that she had met someone who told her she was under threat, this seems to be an example of the effects of a psychotic belief reinforcing itself, an example of confirmation bias. She believed that she had been told that the criminals were about to be released. This interpretation of her meeting is presumably based on her strong belief that this would happen, but the interaction was taken as evidence that the belief which generated the experience is true.

I wasn't really sure what was real and what was delusional interpretation. Certainly, it didn't seem impossible that she could have been seeking out people who had asked her to import drugs 20 years before, and if so, this obviously presented a danger for her. It seemed very unlikely that anyone had gone to prison. On the other hand, this could all be delusion. I didn't know if the house she sought out was the house of the drug dealers or not. Fortunately, no one answered the door. If someone had opened the door Jane would probably have got a negative response. The person answering the door wouldn't have understood what she was talking about and would have possibly felt threatened, or alternately they may have regarded her as mentally ill and called the ambulance. Either way her interpretation of the reaction as a hostile response would be likely to fuel her paranoia.

Second Phase of Therapy

In Jane's case, the initial phase of therapy had not permanently reduced her delusional belief or her fear of the hallucinatory voices that she heard, and she still suffered from almost complete social avoidance based on her persecutory anxieties. She had, however, turned up to her appointments regularly and tolerated the anxieties that came from interacting with another person. So, it would have seemed unhelpful to stop working with her after a short period. We moved into a phase of psychodynamic-influenced psychotherapy. I stopped being as active in the sessions. (After all there are only so many times you can have the same discussion.) I let her talk about whatever was on her mind and I put my energies into to trying to understand and reflect back her feelings. When I linked her current experiences and fears to her childhood experiences and feelings, she was quite able to see the links. But most of the time, I was listening to her and clarifying what she was feeling about what she brought along.

Psychodynamic Conceptualisation

In Jane's case, her delusional system has to a large degree replaced relationships with people in the real world. Much of the time, she is relating to hostile persecuting projections and lives in fear of being killed. Many events in the real world are seen through the lens of her delusional system, so she misinterprets what people say or do in light of this system. Cameron (1959), following Freud (1933), regards the construction of a delusional system as an attempt at restoration—so relating to persecutory figures is at least an attempt to establish a relationship with an "object". This may be preferable to being completely alone. It is an attempt to relate to other people.

The events surrounding the onset of the delusion are important, and an alternative approach to therapy to the one that I took (inspired by some of the modified psychodynamic work described by Bollas, 2015) would be to clarify the events leading up to the onset of her delusion 20 years before and, in particular, her life before the onset of the delusional system. She had lived as an independent adult from some time before the onset of psychosis so to reconnect to this real history as opposed to the mythical history of her persecution by criminals would be an interesting approach to the therapy.

Jane's delusional system seems to a large degree to be a reflection of her childhood world. Her father is a persecuting evil force while Jane and her mother and siblings are helpless victims. Her inner abusive father is projected onto the external world. The delusion represents a return of the internal persecutory object which has now been projected out. The relationship-pattern which was originally based on her relationship with her abusive father was internalised and now returns to haunt her through being projected out into the drug dealers, people she meets on the street and voices that she hears through the wall. She is living in constant fear of being killed as, when she was a child, she lived in fear of her father returning from the pub in a bad violent mood. She did not connect the two and, as she believed that she was really being persecuted, this is obviously not surprising.

Her history of child abuse doesn't, of course, explain the delusional system, because many people have histories of being beaten or abused in other ways who do not develop delusions. On the other hand, it seems likely that these experiences are part of the explanation (because the themes are so closely mirrored). But something has happened to Jane which involves a change in the functioning of her ego. She cannot draw the boundary between her imaginings and reality. She has withdrawn from contact with other people and her world is populated by projections from her unconscious mind. What we can observe more clearly is her current state of mind and her current relationships to others.

When the voices accused her of having abused a child, this seems to also be a repetition with her in the role of her father in her life. She is identified with her father and then accused of having harmed children. The accusation that is made against her could be correctly made against her father. This obviously implies a degree of disintegration of the "boundaries of the ego" and she has no insight into this at all. In her relationship with me, this theme played out too. Obviously, for someone to engage in an hour of psychological therapy once a week, when they see virtually no one else, is in itself an important change in their life. She now had someone that she could talk to about her life and her mind, whereas she had previously been largely isolated, alone with her world of projections (the pseudo-community in Norman Cameron's [1959] language).

At the end of many of our sessions, she left my office and closed the door only to then knock on the door, re-enter, and ask me if I had called her a child abuser. Here while she is with me, she can hold onto the idea of me as a good object but as soon as she is not in my presence, she hears me attacking her. The other version of me is a hostile persecutor. This is an example of the importance of endings in therapy. Here what is useful in the psychodynamic account is that the therapy relationship with me is part of the therapy. If she can develop a positive relationship with me, this is a counter to the idea that all relationships are dangerous and to be retreated from. So, examining her idea that I am one of her voices calling her a child abuser is to work on her problem in a direct way. It's not that this is a behavioural experiment about the voices as illusions. It's really about whether and to what degree she can trust. The most important role of the therapist here, seen in this way, is to persist in being a "good enough object" in contrast to her surrounding persecutory objects, and to avoid being pushed into being either a negative or an idealised role.

It would have made no sense here to suggest any of this to her as an interpretation because, for her, the accusing voices are not symptoms but perceptions, and how can a perception be explained by a memory or an impulse? But I felt that what was helpful about the therapy was first that it was an opportunity to be listened to. She didn't have any other contacts with people in which she was heard. Actually, of course, she had hardly any other contacts at all. Also, as this was a psychological therapy, the conversations we had didn't involve discussions about medication or assessment of her mental state. And these discussions, although important, do tend to take over a meeting and become the only reason for talking.

She would bring along events from her week and we would talk them through. How to deal with difficulties and also the meaning that she put on events? Sometimes she talked about the past, or her sister, and sometimes she began by talking about voices.

I spoke to her a few months after the termination (therapy went on for about two years altogether) to find out how she was doing and she told me that it had been very difficult when the therapy ended. Of course, this wasn't only the end of the therapy relationship but she had few other relationships to replace it with. Another useful input with Jane would have been to try to engage her in community activities or day programmes from clients with mental health problems, but her severe paranoia and anxiety did preclude this type of intervention.

If psychosis is a breakdown in the functioning of the ego associated with a withdrawal from contact with other people, one way to proceed is not only by addressing particular symptoms but also by addressing the underlying difficulty in relating to others by addressing problems in the therapy relationship. In Jane's case, this was her paranoia directed at me, and her grief about the end of the relationship which I hadn't seen (until she told me about it at follow-up). Why, you might wonder, did I miss the importance of the ending of the therapy with Jane? I think that in part this was to do with my focus on her symptoms and working on trying to modify them. I was in a frame of mind in which I was not focusing on Jane as a person but on Jane's symptoms. This is the mistake of the biological psychiatrist. Also, when we disavow the idea of schizophrenia as an illness but focus on symptoms, we can also be blinded by the atomisation involved in this. You can treat someone's "voices" by normalising them as an experience that many people have but lose sight of the connection of the voices to other issues that the person has. The paranoia, withdrawal from contact with others and the delusional system which the voices fit into in Jane's case, can hardly be thought of as a normal psychological situation. That part of someone's thinking could be so alienated from them that think it's someone else voice is really a rather abnormal experience. This is a less reassuring aspect of Jane's situation. In fact, it is terrifying.

In Jane's case, the importance of social withdrawal is clear. Her solitary existence and her paranoid fears fuel each other. Harry Stack Sullivan (1962) tried to treat people with schizophrenia by bringing them into hospital and giving them alcohol in an effort to reduce their anxiety and therefore increase their social interactions, which was an attempt to overcome the paranoid avoidance, such as we see with Jane.

In Jane's case, her delusional beliefs, and the experiences that go along with them, are like memories. It is helpful to hold this aspect of her experiences in mind.

References

Bollas, C. (2015). *When the sun bursts: The enigma of schizophrenia*. New Haven, CT: Yale University Press.

Cameron, N. (1959). The paranoid pseudo-community revisited. *American Journal of Sociology*, *65*(1), 52–58.

Freud, S. (1933). *Introductory lectures on psychoanalysis: New series*. London: Penguin.

Nelson, H. (2005). *Cognitive therapy with delusions and hallucinations*. Cheltenham: Stanley Thornes.

Sullivan, H. S. (1962). *Schizophrenia as a human process*. New York: W.W. Norton.

8 Siobhan

The Fear of Failure—Delusion During Times of Hardship

Siobhan was a 37-year-old woman who came from an Irish background. When I met her, she was living in East London. I saw her at the Psychological Therapies Department at Hackney Hospital. A few years before I saw her, she had been admitted to hospital because she was suicidal and, at that time, had been floridly psychotic. She had thought that her neighbours were using electronic equipment to spy on her all the time and monitor her private conversations. I hadn't read the notes prior to seeing her, but later on I did look at the notes and read the assessment of the inpatient team. She had lived in one room in a shared house. She had recovered from the acute psychosis but had been left with a longstanding delusion about a former work colleague harassing her. This was, she felt, motivated partly by malice and partly by romantic interest.

She had previously been seen in the clinic for over a year by a nurse-therapist who had left the service. After this she had not been taken on by another psychologist or nurse therapist but had been seeing a general psychiatrist for a review once a month. She had not had a case manager and not had any psychological intervention during that time. In the past, in addition to seeing the nurse-therapist, she had attended groups for social anxiety, run by the nurse-therapists. She hadn't found the social anxiety group helpful but she had found the one-to-one counselling supportive.

At our first meeting, she was slightly early for her appointment and smiled when I came to bring her into my office. She explained that she had seen the previous counsellor in the same clinic until she had left. She began talking about her current problems. She was working as a clerk in the local social security office. She found the workplace difficult, mainly because she perceived many of the women that she worked with as hostile and petty. I asked her what was bringing her along and she talked a lot about her work. She took to talking about her problems and her feelings very easily, which may have been partly due to having been in therapy before. She now lived alone in a small one-room flat, rather than in shared accommodation. Living alone seemed to trigger her social anxieties and suspicions less. Her mother lived with Siobhan's sister and her sister's husband. Siobhan saw her family each week. I made some comments about how it must be strange to have

DOI:10.4324/9781003168379-10

a different therapist, and a man to boot, but none of these comments really seemed to jell with her. She explained that it had been difficult after the previous therapist left and she didn't see anyone.

Over the next few sessions, she explained her problems and I took a personal history. As she told me her story, it emerged that she had the longstanding belief that an ex-colleague had been hacking into her computer, leaving messages for her which were usually taunts or verbal attacks of some type. This was a man that she had initially found attractive and she had felt that he returned her affections, but that he didn't do this in a direct way. This contrasted with the fact that she didn't have a partner and that one of her deepest wishes was that she would meet a man and be married.

Her mother and sister lived nearby but her father was in Northern Ireland, and she heard from him infrequently. She remembered her father as a violent man. He had a reputation for being particularly cruel when he had been in the police force. She remembered him being violent towards her mother and also being away for long periods of time, on secret operations. On the other hand, although she was frightened of him, she also felt that he had done an important job in very difficult circumstances, protecting her community in the violent atmosphere of the times. She hadn't experienced any of the political violence herself, but it was there in the background and she remembered soldiers patrolling on the streets and tank traps on the roads into Belfast. However, it wasn't her father or the environment that were most upsetting for her. She said that it was her mother who had been most traumatising for her. She remembered her mother as critical and controlling, and her mother was there all the time, whereas her father was gone for long periods. If anyone outside of the family said anything about Siobhan, her mother would stand up to them and protect her, but she had been persistently critical and controlling of Siobhan herself. Siobhan said, furthermore, her mother didn't teach her how to stand up to others and she felt that her mother had let her down in this. She remembered getting very upset about her mother invalidating her in a variety of ways.

She had been bullied over long periods at school. At secondary school, there was a boy who liked her but, when she wasn't interested in seeing him, he bullied her by making sarcastic remarks about her and her appearance, and he also got the other boys to pick on her. She remembered, at age 15, being asked to read something out in class and then being teased by the other pupils, with the boy who she rebuffed leading the bullying. This was one of the first times that she felt socially anxious.

Her first overdose at 18 was in response to feeling unacceptable and an outsider because of the bullying. She wasn't seriously hurt and went to the emergency department but wasn't admitted. She ended up seeing a minister for pastoral counselling, and she saw him over a number of years. Unfortunately, the minister, who was in his 60s, seduced her and began an affair with her. This was confusing in a number of ways. First he told her that she wanted to have a relationship with him but wasn't aware of her true feelings. He told her that as a counsellor he knew what she truly wanted. This was very confusing and she wasn't sure if he was right or not. After that she wasn't sure of his motives when he gave her advice. For example, when he suggested that she shouldn't see a particular boy she was interested in, she didn't know if that was because the boy was not good for her or if he was acting out of jealousy. He told her that her family were bad for her and she began to distance herself from them which, she now felt, had made her situation far worse. Some of what he said she found helpful, but he was cynical about people and suggested that she should not trust them. He was very negative about boys she met and she thought, looking back, that this was manipulative. The main problem was that this made her confused about her feelings and about other people including her family.

After studying English at University, she had worked as an assistant to a lawyer in Ulster and had done some study in law. She left Northern Ireland to be near her mother, who had gone to London to get away from her father. When Siobhan arrived, she found clerical work in a law firm but she gave this up, because she found it difficult to fit in with the other workers. It was at this time she began to believe that she was being bugged. The evidence for this was mainly feeling that things that turned up on social media referred to her.

After some time, she explained the circumstances around her psychotic breakdown and admission to hospital. She had lived with her family when she first arrived in London but, after an argument, her sister had said that she couldn't live with them any longer. She had gone back to live with her father in Belfast but then came back to London and lived on her own in shared accommodation. This was when she got the job with the law firm. Her account of the conflict with her sister was that she (Siobhan) had complained about the cleanliness of the house and her sister became angry about this, and that she had been assaulted by her sister during the ensuing argument. Siobhan contacted the police who weren't able to act on her accusation, as no one in the family was going to back up her accusation, but her sister had then said that she was no longer welcome in the house and Siobhan had left that night.

There are a number of themes running through the history she gave. First, there is a theme of bullying. Her father bullied her mother and her mother bullied Siobhan. She was bullied by her co-worker. This is linked to her social anxiety. Her anxiety about other people is that they will put her down or judge her and she will not be able to defend herself. The relationship with the Minister was an example of having her trust broken and of other people being manipulative and deceitful—out for what they can get. She had mixed feelings about the Minister at the time, feeling that he was sometimes helpful, but that at times feeling that he was manipulating her for his own purposes in a Svengali like way. He could make her doubt her own feelings. This not knowing what to believe, or which people to trust, seems to link to her later delusional idea about feeling that other people have sinister hidden motives. Her delusion about her co-worker seems a repetition of her feelings about the Minister, in that she has ambivalent feelings and she cannot be sure that people are not scheming against her. There is a theme of ambivalence in her close relationships. The minister sometimes gave her helpful advice but manipulated her into a sexual relationship, and in other ways, she was attracted to her ex-colleague but he was harassing her, the boy at school who found her attractive promoted a campaign of bullying against her and her mother protected her but was critical and controlling.

The Therapy

Therapy began with a long period of engagement of several months. She was in therapy with me for about three years altogether. Siobhan was distressed by her delusion at the beginning of therapy. She found having her computer hacked intrusive, but she felt that her ex-colleague's eventual aim was to have her as his wife. At one point in the therapy, I raised the possibility of examining the truth of this belief, but Siobhan did not think that this would be worthwhile so we never did address the delusion in this direct way (although we did address the delusion in an indirect way as explained later). The delusional belief had some unacknowledged advantages for her. Although she found it annoying, it also meant that someone was interested in her.

At the beginning, I spent several months listening to Siobhan and developing trust. Most of her pressing concerns were to do with her social anxiety, and with her relationships with men. She hadn't had a partner since her teens and finding a relationship in which she was happy was her primary ambition. She had a low opinion of people in general and wasn't very interested in cultivating friends, rather what she deeply desired was a husband.

We began to work on her social anxiety and on getting her a job, using exposure and role play. I explained the cognitive model of social anxiety. Being anxious in a social situation made her focus on negative cues and to not notice positive cues. It made her interpret cues in a more negative and threatening way than was justified by the evidence. Furthermore, the anxiety affected her ability to interact with other people and to listen and think clearly about what they are saying. I suggested a graded exposure programme. If she could enter social situations repeatedly and frequently, her anxiety would probably reduce. In general, she didn't feel anxious at work anymore and I suggested that this was likely to be due to repeatedly going to work, so that it demonstrated how the approach can work for her.

I will now present the details of some sessions, to illustrate the use of the therapy relationship in her case.

A Session

She explained that she was having a problem at work. There was another worker who was deliberately invading her personal space and making her uncomfortable by standing too close to her. She doesn't want to talk to him. He has dark skin. She doesn't find dark skin attractive. She likes fair skin and blue eyes. She wasn't sure what to do about the man at work. She said that she knew that she didn't like him standing close to her and that he did it as a provocation. This annoyed her more.

This is a situation that is quite common in dealing with psychotic clients. This belief (that another worker had realised that she didn't like him to stand close to her and had then done it deliberately) is obviously not bizarre. It could, of course, be true. On the other hand, it could be a reflection of her tendency to interpret other people's motives as hostile. Or it could have begun as her perception and then generated the feared reaction, by the other worker detecting her feelings towards him. Her hostile feelings towards the co-worker affect her behaviour towards him and her perception of him and result in him playing into the dysfunctional complementary role pair (in CAT terms) or projective identification in psychodynamic terms.

I clarified what she felt had happened and that she felt he had done this maliciously. (This links to her delusion about the ex-colleague except that in the previous case she had been attracted to him, and now it was reversed. In both cases, she felt that there was an attraction between her and a man but that this ended up with her being harassed and intruded upon. In both cases, someone is attracted to someone and is rebuffed.) Her anxiety about the work colleague is not delusional, but it is on the same theme and springs from the same psychological roots. Her anxiety about being intruded upon by men obviously links to her past experience with the minister and earlier to her relationship to her father (who she saw as a powerful, dangerous man). Here there is a victim–abuser reciprocal role pair, in cognitive analytic therapy terms.

She had gone on to complain to her manager about her colleague invading her personal space. The manager responded to this by reviewing the video from the CCTV of her interacting with the co-worker. Her manager said that she couldn't see anything that looked inappropriate and also raised it with the co-worker. Now the roles shift and he is being watched on camera and investigated. He had apparently become angry and had made complaints about her unfriendliness. This seems to be an example of how a suspicious belief can act as a self-fulfilling prophecy, as Norman Cameron (1959) has described. Siobhan firmly believed that the colleague had been persecuting her. Her persecutory feelings are directly affecting her life problems, so it would be good to be able to intervene with a cognitive intervention to investigate whether her perception of the current situation as persecutory was correct. However, this did not seem to be likely to be helpful. In the current conflict I thought that she would take any direct expression of doubt about her belief as an invalidation and siding with her persecutors. Therefore, I took it up with her in relation to how helpful her belief was rather than whether she was right about what had happened. Was it useful to act in a particular way? What was a professional way to act given that she had to share a working space with him?

This particular conflict at work does reflect on the client's relationship to the therapist. The relationship with me was idealised. I was the helpful (not to say blue eyed and pale) object in contrast to the bad rapacious co-worker. Again, it did not seem helpful here to raise this with the client directly. But it did seem important to be aware of this so avoid, inter alia, acting this particular idealisation out.

Transcripts of Sessions

In the following transcripts of some sessions with Siobhan, I want to illustrate how paranoid themes present in the material she brings to session. Mainly these are not frankly delusional, but they are related themes. Allowing her to talk about whatever problem is on her mind is obviously taken from the analytic method, although I am far more active than most analytic therapists and more forthcoming with my opinions.

The previous session had to be cancelled due to a problem with the internet connection.

Client:	It has been good since I saw you last. There haven't been any problems at work or at home.
Therapist:	How did the exam go?
Client:	Oh I haven't seen you? After our session I did the exam online but there were problems with the internet, so I called them up and they are going to reschedule the exam.
Therapist:	Oh. That's a shame.
Clint:	Yes. Also, I've decided to drop one of the courses. It's really hard. I had a look at the exam questions. They are multiple choice but really difficult.
Therapist:	Oh I see. So, did you want to talk about that or was there something in particular that you would like to focus on today?
Client:	Still my social anxiety.
Therapist:	Ok. Was there a time recently . . .?
Client:	(pause). I can't think of an example. I don't think there was a bad example. I'm anxious all the time.
Therapist:	Maybe you don't have any bad examples because you avoid situations that make you anxious.
Client:	Yes. Probably. I can't think of a situation in particular but it's around whenever I am with people really. Oh, there was one

occasion with my brother-in-law. They came around. And we had a visitor who was asking me about my job. I said it was ok and Ann was saying that I am the boss's right hand.

Therapist: Sorry?

Client: That the boss favoured me. When he had gone, she asked me "Why didn't you say more about your job to him?" and I said "Well what did you want me to say?" and she said "Oh yes. I used to be shy but I got over it. You should put yourself forward"

Therapist: And what did you say?

Client: I didn't say anything. I felt really anxious. She was also saying about me that I always give someone a present when they have given me a present, that I'm good at fulfilling my duties. But that isn't why I give presents. I don't do it because it's a duty.

Therapist: You don't return presents because it says that you should in some rule book but because you want to. It comes from your heart.

Client: Yes.

Therapist: So in these examples Ann tells you what to do or implies that your motives for doing things are not good ones.

Client: Yes.

Therapist: So what is the worst thing about her saying these things? Are you bothered by her not liking you?

Client: Well. I'm not really bothered about what she thinks about me.

Therapist: You aren't worried about her opinion of you?

Client: No.

Therapist: If she met me and had a bad opinion of me you wouldn't think less of me?

Client: No! (Laughs)

Therapist: So what is it about this that makes you feel anxious?

Client: Well I think that it's because it reminds me of my mother.

Therapist: In the past?

Client: Well now as well, but she has always been like this. And you know that thing I was talking about Ann? Where she indirectly puts people down?

Therapist: Yes.

Client: Well my mother does that too.

Therapist: Yes. Is there a time you can think of in the past when you had the same feelings that you had with Ann the other day?

Client: (pause) I was with my mother and Shelia (Siobhan's sister). Sheila had noticed how my mother had been with me, telling me what to do and criticising me and she had started to do the same thing.

Therapist: How old were you at the time?

Client: About 15. Sheila began to say critical things to me. And I got upset. I stood up and I picked up the ash tray and I held it really hard in both my hands, like this (she demonstrates holding her arms straight out with her fingers of both hands pointing at each other). I shouted "Stop it".

Therapist: And then what did you do?

Client: I left the room.

Therapist: And what were your feelings in this episode.

Client: Oh I felt upset and anxious.

Therapist: And powerless?

Client: Yes.

Therapist: So this feeling is the same as the feeling you get these days, for example with Ann, where you feel someone is putting you down and you feel defenceless. So, are you ok to do some imagery around this event?

Client: Yes.

Therapist: Ok. If you would like to close your eyes and try to picture the event with your mother and Ann. Can you do that?

Client: Yes.

Therapist: What is going on?

Client: I am sitting with my mother and Sheila and she has been saying nasty things to me and I get up. And I'm feeling really upset and I'm shouting "Stop it" and then I run out of the room.

Therapist: Does anyone come with you?

Client: No.

Therapist: Ok so let's follow you out. Where did you go when this happened?

Client: I can't remember.

Therapist: Lets imagine you go into a room. What can you see?

Client: I can see me crying.

Therapist: What do you want to say to you at fifteen?

Client: I want to tell her that it isn't her fault.

Therapist: Ok. Go ahead and tell her.

Client: "It's not your fault"

Therapist: (To the imagined chid) It's not your fault, you didn't do anything wrong. It's just your family aren't treating you right. (To the adult client) What do you want to do now?

Client: I want to put my arm around her.

Therapist: Ok. Go ahead and do that. And now ask 15-year-old you if she will be alright.

Client: I won't be alright.

Therapist: Ask her what she wants.

Client: I want to get out of there. I know what she has to put up with for all those years.

Therapist: Ok. Let's you and I take her out. We go out into our car. You sit in the back with her and I'll drive. Where shall we take her?

Client: Somewhere safe.

Therapist: Did you have any relatives?

Client:	No.
Therapist:	How about we take her to a safe house while we work it out?
Client:	Ok.
Therapist:	And how is she going?
Client:	Good. She is cuddling up to me.
Therapist:	Ok. If you would like to open your eyes. How did you find that?
Client:	It was good. I feel a lot of relief.
Therapist:	So this is what comes up when you get socially anxious and we have to try to reassure and comfort the fifteen-year-old you. Actually, it's not so much, for example, Ann, that bothers you, it's more the part of you that joins in.
Client:	I have an inner bully.
Therapist:	Yes and that's what we need to work on together.
Therapist:	It's nearly time now. How did you find the session today?
Client:	Yes it was good. Although I feel a bit exhausted and deflated now.
Therapist:	Why do you think that is?
Client:	Well it was exhausting remembering and getting upset about it.
Therapist:	Yes, it's a sad memory and we are trying to fight this inner bully but you have to remember some of these things in order to do that. Will you let me know next time how you are after the session please?
Client:	Yes sure.

Commentary on This Session

In this session, the client and I work on a particular aspect of her social anxiety—the inner critic or bully, or the inner persecutory object and her relationship to it. There is the role play in which I try to coach her to deal with her inner critical mother in a more assertive way, or as in this example, to make her feel that she is not all alone in this and that what happened to her in the past was (by inference) wrong and that she should have been protected from it. However, there is another perspective on this role paly, which is that the client trusts me to solve this problem for her. I am presenting myself as trustworthy and she and I collaborate in dealing with the problem in imagination. During the role paly, she feels validated and she says that she felt relief from imagining the situation in a changed way. The hope is that in current social situations, she will be able to stand up more to the inner bully, over a period of time, of course. This seems to have been helpful in her case in this session. However, there is also a down side to this, which is having to remember the situation. What doesn't emerge in the therapy when the therapist imposes a structure like this (the therapist as a good and helpful person who can be supportive and give good guidance) is the negative feelings that the client may have towards the therapist. These feelings may be explicit or they may be unarticulated, but the focus on the role play drives them out of the therapy room. There is also another danger here which is that this procedure may well encourage idealisation of the therapist, by excluding the client's negative feelings about the therapist from the relationship. A psychoanalyst might argue that this was a very good reason for not using this type of role play with psychotic clients (or indeed anyone else).

Alternatively, when using role play, one can keep the danger of idealisation in mind, and the possibility of negative feelings towards the therapist and deal with these when they arise. For example, in a previous role play between the client and the minister, I had asked her what she would like her and me to do in the imagery once we had left the psychiatrists office. She had said that she didn't want to go anywhere and I had felt that she was anxious about her and me getting closer in the imagined scene than she would be comfortable with. So, I had suggested that I might drop her off at home.

A Later Session

Some months later in her fortnightly sessions, Siobhan wanted to focus more on her social anxiety, and then on completing her diploma course. This was important as she had been in a more senior role in Ulster than she was in England, and she thought the diploma in legal secretarial studies would help her to find work. She didn't really like her job in the call centre and wanted to get back to the role she had had in Northern Ireland. She felt that if she didn't finish the course and qualify, she was wasting all the time that she had spent studying earlier on. She studied at night when she got home from work. Another pressing goal was to reduce her social anxiety, which limited her interactions with others and also made interviews very difficult. She had applied for a post in legal aid but had been rejected after she had had a recorded automated video interview. It seemed that she had given very short answers during the interview as she had felt anxious. She had taken a course to help her present well in interviews which had included some coaching on interview practice. She had never taken this up so she was still entitled to this free interview practice. She had also decided in the session that as she was not completing her homework for her course, she would contact the university and ask to postpone the current course she was taking until the next semester. At the following session, she hadn't completed these actions and we had a discussion about this as well as a number of other things.

The session I reproduce here was the session following that.

The Next Session

I continued to see her on Zoom. The internet connection was not good and I was concerned that we might have to reschedule the session.

Client:	There is something I wanted to talk about from last time; something that you said.
Therapist:	Ok. What was that?
Client:	Last session when we were talking about the diploma work and the interview practice and you said that I was good at procrastinating, and I felt that you sounded a bit like my mother.
Therapist:	What did I say?
Client:	We were talking about how I hadn't booked into the interview practice classes and you said I was good at procrastinating, and we both laughed but I felt upset. It was like being with my previous psychologist.
Therapist:	Well I'm sorry I said that. I understand why you put things off.
Client:	I felt "Here we go again", and I was thinking about how I would have to find another psychologist and how when I did, they would probably let me down so that wherever I went I would just get let down, so what was the point?
Therapist:	And how long were you thinking that?
Client:	Well at first, I wasn't going to come back, but then I calmed down after a day or two and decided to come. And I have told you.
Therapist:	Yes. Well, I'm glad you were able to come back and let me know. I understand that you put things off because they make you very uncomfortable and anxious. In the longer-term putting things, off doesn't get you what you want or need but in the short term it works.
Client:	It was more intense with the other psychologist. I kept saying that I needed to come and she was quite cold and just kept repeating that it wasn't possible due to a change in how they worked. And I was crying and she was just really cold with me. I felt that you couldn't be trusted, but then I thought it's not what I usually expect from you so I decided to come along.
Therapist:	I'm glad you did. And feeling criticised has a history with you.
Client:	I was thinking that it would always be the same with any psychologist and I would be on my own.
Therapist:	I think that you felt like I just wanted to criticise you. The idea that you had of me before just sort of disappeared.
Client:	Yes.
Therapist:	Did you think of ringing me up?
Client:	No.
Therapist:	You can ring me if there is something like this that is making you think of not coming back.
Client:	I don't want to ring up. I like that we don't talk outside of the session. If we talked out of the session it would remind me of the minister I used to see.

Therapist: Can you say a bit more about that?

Client: Talking to you outside of the session makes me nervous because of what happened with him.

Therapist: You are anxious that something like that could happen again here?

Client: I don't think that you would do that.

Therapist: Maybe you get anxious about what you might do?

Client: I don't think that you or me are going to do anything like that. It's like a phobia though.

Therapist: Because of what happened it's important to have the clear rules around when we meet and don't meet.

Client: Yes. He did me a lot of damage. You know he taught me to lie? When I first saw him the first thing he told me was that I shouldn't tell anyone in my family about what happened in counselling. He was preparing me. And I couldn't tell anyone. My mother is so conservative you know? I told one of my friends and she blamed me for it. She said that I shouldn't have gone along with it. You know the first time he kissed me. There was a bird in his office and he said "look at the bird" and while I looked at the bird, he kissed me. I was shocked and he said, "What's the matter I kiss all my female friends?" Do you know I told him about having been interfered with as a child? Not by anyone in my family but by people outside the family.

Therapist: Adults?

Client: Yes by adults. And he said that he didn't know why I was getting so upset. His patients that had been molested as children or raped told him that they enjoyed it. Can you imagine? Women being terrified and then he says that they enjoyed it? I began to wonder "Did I enjoy that?" It made me doubt myself.

Therapist: He took advantage of you in the counselling and then he made you doubt what you thought you knew and felt about your feelings. This was really very damaging.

Client: Yes, I had the issues with my family so I went to him and he just made it worse.

I told him that I would report him to the Church board. He said "Go ahead. I will tell them that you are delusional". I did contact the board but they never got back to me. If my father found out he would kill him, or at least he might attack him, and then I don't want that to happen to my father. Still, I found out that he has got lung cancer and he is dying.

Commentary

The session opens with an accusation that I was condescending and critical in the previous session, and that she had had to stop seeing a previous psychologist because they turned out to be uncaring. It is an indication of how fragile the situation is. She hopes for an idealised good object but is continually disappointed and if there is any sense that the person that she is relating to has any faults they fall off the pedestal and become a bad object. However, she returns, and this allows me the chance to deal with the persecutory fear in the moment and is an example of the usefulness of negative transference. Later she talks of being seduced by a minister in her church and the damage done by this. She talks about this when I have suggested that she can ring me outside of the session and although she denies that she is worried about my intentions consciously she likes the rigid boundaries of the sessions as it makes her feel safe. Although she doesn't acknowledge this, it seems likely that she fears getting closer to me. It's important here not to contradict the client about her accusation towards me. There is often some truth in the accusation and it is important that the client feels that this has been heard. The other important aspect of this session is that the client spontaneously mentions that the rigid boundaries around the counselling allow her to feel safer in the interaction.

The inner bad object (which has been projected into the men that were trying to harass her by hacking into her Facebook or planting cameras in the room) was projected into the previous psychologist when she had mentioned termination, and then projected into me. The most important thing here is how to react to her perception. Not insisting that that she misperceived my intention and not over apologising, but to continue to see her and take her perception as another thing to talk about.

A Later Session

Siobhan began by saying that she had had a problem with a friend at work but she didn't want to spend the session talking about this problem as it had been resolved. She had something to tell me. She had signed up for a course in creative writing. This was a course through a technical college. It only involved one hour a week. And what she wanted to write about was the minister. The course was on line so she would not have to meet with the other participants. What did I think? I said that this seemed like a great idea. I said that the one hour a week seemed much more achievable than the previous two or three hours a night of the secretarial studies. I said that this seemed particularly difficult, as she had hated the secretarial studies. Of course, she would need to think about how confidential the writing would be and whether she would be expected to share it with people other than the course tutor. She said that she wouldn't want to share this with anyone apart from the course tutor and me. She went on to ask me why I thought she couldn't get a job. She was applying for jobs in administration and customer service but she wasn't getting interviews. Did I think that this was to do with her being Irish? But there were lots of people from Northern Ireland employed in public services. Was it that she was incompetent? I asked her what other possible explanations there were. She looked a bit lost and said that she couldn't think of any. I said that maybe it was difficult to get work in general. What factors made it hard to get work, did she think? She said that she wasn't sure, so I suggested that possibly if there are a lot of applicants for a job, they have to come up with a simple way of reducing the number of people to interview and that one way was, for example, to only interview people who had relevant experience in an area. I said that the idea that people were biased against her because of being from Northern Ireland could be a poisonous idea, not because no one was prejudiced, but because it was difficult to know if they were and that, because of that, any slight or rejection could be seen as an indication of prejudice. She thought about this but didn't reply. Then she said that the psychiatrist had prescribed the beta-blockers for her to reduce her anxiety at her next interview, and she had now got the prescription filled. She could test out the tablet when an interview came up. She said that I had suggested that she should try to exercise even for a very short time and that what she had done was to start using the exercise bike. Finally, she returned to writing up the memoir about the minister and she said that the confidentiality was important. If people from her community knew about what had happened, they would blame her. Her sister blamed her for what had happened. I asked her how she knew this. She said that in the middle of an argument, she had said so.

Commentary on the Session

In this session, she has given up the rigid demands of insisting that she should complete her exams and had chosen two goals for herself. She had adapted my suggestion (to exercise for a short period) to one that she felt more ownership of, and she had found a course which would not be demanding a goal but that would fit in with her own interests (writing) and which was achievable (writing a memoire rather than a novel). There is no feeling of clinical paranoia around any of this. She wonders if she isn't getting a job because of prejudice. But, of course, this is possibly true so it would be wrong to think of this persecutory idea as delusional. The most noticeable change, however, is that she is choosing things to do because she wants to do them, rather than because, for example, her sister had suggested it or it would be good for her capacity to earn money. At the end of the session, I asked if she had thought about what she would want if the possibility of seeing each other via Zoom stopped (which had been suggested recently in the press). She said that she hadn't thought about this and we ended without a conclusion about what she would do. It is noticeable in these later sessions that she talked about her delusion less often. One hypothesis is that her preoccupation with her delusional belief decreased as she engaged in the relationship with the therapist.

A Later Session

Later in the therapy, she had gone for an interview in which she had had to role play with other candidates. She had surprised herself as she thought that she had done well at the interview despite being nervous. Unfortunately, she was unsuccessful. When she found out that she hadn't got the job the old ideas about having her computer hacked into by her old work colleague returned. The delusion is to the front of her mind when she is being frustrated by life. It is an unsignalled metaphor for her feelings about her life and the frustrations that she keeps running into. Her delusion symbolises, amongst other things, her experience of the world as harsh and uncaring.

General Comments

Generally, the feeling in the sessions is positive and relaxed and she enjoys coming to the meetings. There are two occasions when the possibility of a negative response to me occurs. One is the occasion in the transcript when she takes offence at my comment about her procrastination, the other occurred fairly early in the therapy. She had been in the waiting room and I emerged with another psychologist who had been having supervision with me. As we came out of my office, we had been laughing about something. When she came into the office, she asked me if we had been talking about her. I simply said that we hadn't. Apart from these two occasions the atmosphere was generally positive, and she valued the opportunity to talk. She expressed no interest in having friends and she was not on good terms with her relatives, but wanted to find a partner and find more rewarding work. The main problem that she presents in the sessions is anxiety in social situations. Her heightened sensitivity to possible hostility in others has led her to withdraw from other people and a lack of pleasure in anything. And although she would like a partner, she also feels that she doesn't want a partner as it always goes wrong. The belief about being spied upon recurred at times when things were going wrong (as in the example when she didn't succeed the job interview). She just found the thoughts preoccupied her more and then she noticed examples of odd things going on.

I am an idealised object, and outside of therapy mainly she comes into contact with persecutory objects. When she is unwell this becomes frankly delusional, and other people are perceived as her inner persecutory objects, with little input from their actual personal characteristics. The primary aim of the therapy is to establish a good object in her external world which may then be internalised. The main threat to this is that I am idealised and badness is kept out of the room. I mean because I am idealised the relationship is to some degree brittle and in danger of failing. This approach seems compatible with also working on the symptoms that she does bring, such as social anxiety. Offering suggestions about strategies or techniques to deal with anxiety or using imagery to rescript a traumatic scene don't seem to disrupt the establishment of the therapist as a good object. An important use of this conceptualisation is to be aware of being either idealised or denigrated in the sessions and to address it.

Reference

Cameron, N. (1959). The paranoid pseudo-community revisited. *American Journal of Sociology*, *65*(1), 52–58.

9 Tom and June

Psychosis in DBT

Tom was referred to the City and Hackney Psychotherapy Department by his Consultant Psychiatrist. He was 23 years old, from a Greek background and there was uncertainty about his diagnosis. He had been diagnosed as having a personality disorder but there was some thought that he might have a bipolar disorder. In the end, many years after I stopped seeing him, the consensus was that he had schizoaffective disorder. He was a slightly built young man with short cut bleached hair. The community mental health team had treated him as having borderline personality disorder and had put him in the DBT programme but this therapy hadn't gone well, and the psychiatrist was unsure if personality disorder was the correct diagnosis, so he was referred to the psychotherapy department for cognitive therapy. He had had a number of impulsive overdoses over the past few years. He also behaved impulsively and sometimes was confused about his identity (e.g. at times he had not been sure if he was gay or straight), and his goals and values could change quickly and dramatically. He also had periods when his mood seemed to be elevated for a longer period of time. I include him in this case series, because he was delusional for six months.

When I met him for an initial assessment, he told me that the problems that he had had with impulsivity and anger were now solved and that his only remaining problem was that he became anxious in some situations. He was now engaged to be married to a young woman who was the same age as him but of a contrasting character. He had been seeing her for some time and seemed very settled. Tom had just begun studying marketing at university and this was going quite well. I began to see him on a weekly basis to work on his goal of reducing his anxiety. He had a lot of friends that he spent time with but didn't have any close friends apart from his partner. He had seen a number of psychologists before doing DBT.

He was the youngest of two children. He had an older brother who struggled with academic study. His parents were unhappily married. His father was a successful businessman and his mother didn't need to work. His father had had a number of affairs and was often away from home. There was always conflict between his parents and Tom sided with his mother whereas his brother sided with his father. Tom had not conformed with his father's

DOI:10.4324/9781003168379-11

traditional ideas about being a man and he felt that his father disapproved of him because of this. His father was very negative about him, and this continued to the present day.

When Tom was around 10 or 11, his mother had developed depression and had been hospitalised for the best part of six months. During this period, he saw a lot of his father, and his father had been critical about everything that he did. His father had taken out his frustrations (about having to be at home to look after the children while his wife was in hospital) on the children. During secondary school, while he was coping with the conflict with his father, he struggled to fit in. He had had a group of friends who had in common that they were disaffected. Since then, he had had many short-term relationships with girls. He later told me that as soon as he felt that there was a problem in a relationship, he ended it before the girl got a chance to end it with him. His admissions to hospital came after overdoses, or threatened overdoses.

More recently, however, he had been with a steady girlfriend and they were engaged to be married. One feature of working with Tom was that at different points in the therapy he presented very differently. So, in the first phase, he was not self-harming and his goals were to study and settle down. The main problems that he brought along during this period were feelings of anxiety, mainly worry and sometimes panic, and his difficulties in his relationship with his parents. His father had been very critical and would tell him he was worthless and would never amount to anything. Now he became angry and abusive towards his parents. He also was continually feeling that he should intervene in arguments between his parents. In contrast, his relationship with his girlfriend was calm and stable. It became clear that his problems were not limited to symptoms of anxiety (which is what he had said at the initial meetings) and that impulsive anger, fear of abandonment, and low self-esteem were all important problems in his life. He was able to turn a blind eye to problems and feelings very effectively. This unfortunately meant that he was often out of touch with his feelings, goals, and problems. His hospital admissions were usually around feelings of wanting to die. Generally, he liked being on the ward, and saw his consultant psychiatrist more often. This raised the possibility that being admitted to the ward was rewarding for him.

After an initial period of therapy focused on anxiety symptoms and family problems, he began to self-harm again. He was in continual conflict with his parents. Shortly after this I began to see him using DBT again. He began attending the skills groups and I became his DBT individual therapist, and structured our individual therapy along the lines of DBT, prioritising thoughts and acts of self-harm in the sessions. He had begun to repeatedly attend the emergency department again and was often admitted, threatening suicide. This was usually precipitated by the conflict at home. He decided to move out and live independently. He moved into a shared house. However, living with strangers made him anxious almost all the time. In his sessions with me, we worked on his anxiety using cognitive and behavioural strategies, but with little effect. In truth, it was difficult to get him to see the worry as unreasonable. After a couple of months, he gave up and moved back in with his parents.

His father disapproved of his course of study, and his life style, but he mainly heard about this through his mother or through other people who saw his father. His father was involved and supportive of his brother.

His difficulty in moving out demonstrated something important about his anger and his relationship with his parents. He clearly had an ambivalent relationship with them, and in particular his father. Although when he lived with him, he was full of anger and hatred for his father, when he lived alone, he felt that he was unable to look after himself and feared being rejected by other people. Here it seems that he has carried over his expectations of his father to the flatmates. In cognitive analytic therapy terms, he has internalised a reciprocal role of Abuser and Victim. He internalised this as a child with his father in the abuser role, and he was in the victimised child role. This reciprocal role pair is dysfunctional not only because it is negative but also because it is black or white. In psychoanalytic theory, this is at bottom a defensive strategy, but however that may be, the pattern is quite clear in Tom's case.

For the first 18 months, the atmosphere in our sessions was calm, although his problems outside continued in much the same way. He began to be admitted to the ward more often and it did seem possible that he had begun to adopt the ward as a second home, and one that was calmer and more supportive, although the level of acuity in the wards in Hackney at this time was very high. He began to become provocative in our sessions, and this did have the advantage of being more alive. At the beginning of one session, he came with a container full of anti-psychotics which he said he was going to take, in the room. Talking with him about why he had come to the session with the tablets didn't get very far, so I ended up walking him to the emergency department. At another session he was talking about a problem with his fiancée and he began to bang the back of his head against the wall. I said that he couldn't do that and he looked at me and asked me who I was to tell him what to do.

Psychotic Developments

In contrast to the settled picture that he presented when first referred when he was later admitted to hospital, he became delusional and this continued for six months. He began to believe that there was a conspiracy originating in the Government to find him out, that he had defrauded the social security and that he was being investigated to be prosecuted for various crimes. If he watched the news, he would believe that he was responsible for all the crime and bad things that were reported. Once he started to believe that he was responsible for some crime he would begin to have "memories" of having committed the crime. So, his solution was to avoid the news on the TV by sitting outside when the news was on.

How does the delusion relate to his other problems? Tom's delusion was based on a number of sources. First, the intuition that news stories related to him, and this intuition became delusional as he believed this with no doubts. One explanation here is that he feels unconscious guilt about how he has behaved towards others and that this guilt has produced the ideas of reference around the news programme. He didn't report feeling guilt about his life, but the guilt can be seen as projected out into other people. Furthermore, this is persecutory guilt. The internalised punishing parent is attacking him with accusations of having committed terrible crimes for which he should be punished. Although he behaved aggressively towards his parents, he felt that they deserved it because of how they had treated him. Again, when he talked about his life, he saw himself, with some jus-tification, as the victim. However, he could turn this around so he could play either end of the reciprocal role. As when he shouted at his father or mother and smashed the house up. The general theme in relationships was of him being either the victim or the abuser. I thought that here the delusion also acted out a particular type of object relations. Having been bullied and treated with distain made it more difficult for him to see the hostility in his own actions. As he is not aware of the cause of the guilt, he finds explanation for it in the news stories reported on the TV. An important part of this explanation is the lack of guilt he expressed about his own actions.

The delusional explanation that he remembers being guilty for the crimes he hears is not bizarre in itself, although when all of the occasions are put together it becomes more bizarre. However, he doesn't have any sense of the unlikeliness of him being responsible for all the crimes mentioned on the news every day. His sense of guilt is split off and attached to crimes that he hears about rather than to his actions. This involves a considerable degree of turning away from reality. Feeling guilty is replaced by feeling responsible for other crimes which were not personal so were not about his relation-ships. His childhood experiences contributed to this. He internalised the unhappy relationship between his parents, and his father's absence led to him internalising an uncaring, disinterested parent. He felt unloved and ignored by his father and not protected from this by his mother.

Precis of Some Sessions

I reproduce in the following a series of sessions that occurred while he was delusional and just after that period. He had been admitted to hospital while he was acutely psychotic and these sessions are from when he was beginning to get some home leave and then at up to six months post discharge from hospital. In all these sessions, his prevailing mood is anxiety.

Session One

This session was while Tom was still on the ward, but had been given home leave. He had been in hospital for two months. He looked a little on edge as he looked around the office and the ward. He began by saying that he had been having unpleasant side effects from one of the drugs he was taking. The psychiatrists were considering giving him Clozapine if this current medication didn't help. It was clear in the way that he said this that he was considerably anxious about this possibility. He went on to talk about his home leave. He said that when he had been at home there had been a visitor who was a friend of his father's. The visitor had talked all the time about politics and the Government. Tom had found this very difficult. He had thought that the visitor was there to give him a warning. I had asked if the visitor had come to be helpful and Tom said that he hadn't felt it was helpful, more threatening. He had come as a message. Also, he had been finding his name in word puzzles that he had been doing, which he felt was strange and significant. It had been so bad that he had had to go back to avoiding the television, as he would hear references to himself all the time. He said he had been unsettled by these events and that it was a sign that he was getting worse. I said that one part of him felt that he was in danger and that people were sending him messages in the form of visitors or hidden in a word puzzle book, while another part of him felt that this was a sign that he was ill. He didn't respond to this but went on to say that he hated hospital, but felt that he couldn't cope outside at home so that there wasn't a solution. He went on to say that his father and he didn't get on and being around him made him angry and anxious. I asked for an example and he had said that he had talked to his father who had said that psychiatrists can have a vested interest in particular medications and that he shouldn't be too trusting. He said that his father saying this just made him worse, and there wasn't anything he could do about this. He felt unable to cope. When on leave he saw a manager reprimanding an employee and he knew if it had been him he would have been unable to cope with the reprimands. He feels incompetent and unable to cope as an adult. I reflected that it seemed an insoluble problem. He didn't want to be in hospital, but felt he couldn't cope outside.

Commentary

In this session, I do not attempt to address the delusional belief, as the overall main problem here seems to be his self-doubt and feeling of inferiority. The delusional belief seems to stem from these feelings which are being precipitated by the environment. He is clearly distressed by the delusion but this is not a chronic delusion which is the stable cause of his distress, but rather seems to be an outcome of feeling highly anxious and with no external support. He has regressed and he is preoccupied by his inner persecutory objects in this session, which are projected out into the Government, Tony Blair or some other agency. He didn't engage me in eye contact for most of the session and I felt as if I were an observer to a dialogue with himself. The visitor at his parents' house is seen as a part of his persecutory world, and not really as a real person. I am shut out in the session. The information from the transference is important here. That is, that I feel as if I scarcely matter to the client, even though I have been seeing him weekly for over a year at this point. This detachment from me is a part of the state of mind that he is in, withdrawn from the real people around him and engaged with his inner world. His relationship to me, his relationship to the feared persecutors, and his relationship to his father are all the same. The important thing during a crisis such as this seems to be to maintain a dialogue and to do this mainly by listening. Any attempt to reduce his distress by examining the truth of the delusion is likely to be counterproductive as it would miss the point that his feelings of being under threat seem primary here and that the most important thing is to keep him engaged. Of course, working on coping skills could also be useful here—maybe DBT's Distress Tolerance skills could help. The theme of the delusion, however, is a theme which is already present in his personal life. The delusion is a symbol of his feelings about his parents when he was a child and the biggest problem he currently struggles with is how to deal with them in a way that isn't destructive.

A Later Session

He had been discharged from hospital. Everywhere he goes, all he hears are people talking about the government. I said that he was out of hospital but feeling very unsafe. He said that he was having panic attacks because of it. I asked how sure he was that the government were monitoring him and he said about 50%. He is trying various things to cope with these experiences, but it keeps recurring. On Facebook, he feels what he writes is monitored by the Government. He doesn't want to tell the psychiatrist or the nurse, as they would increase his Clozapine. I said that he has been feeling increasingly anxious and suspicious and feels threatened a lot of the time, and that this has happened several times since we have been working together. He apologised. I asked him if he felt I was criticising him, and he said that he did. I reflected that he felt that he was with a psychologist who was judging him for not meeting his standards. And he said that he did think that. (So, my reflection on this didn't alleviate this anxiety.) He moved on and told me that he and his girlfriend were going away for the weekend to celebrate their anniversary. He said that the previous year he had felt that he couldn't control his thoughts and this had led to him feeling that someone else was controlling them instead. I asked him what the worst thing would be about these ideas (about the Government monitoring him and controlling his thoughts) being true. He said that he wasn't sure—maybe going to prison. He then asked me whether what he said to me was confidential.

I explained that in general it was. He then became distressed and talked about his fear that he had defrauded the social security by making a false declaration. I asked him what evidence he had and he said that he had a memory of lying on the form. On the other hand, if he had done it, he thinks that he would have been worried about it at the time, and he didn't remember that. I said that I thought that he felt anxious and that the anxiety looked around for something to latch onto—maybe the Government is watching you, maybe you have committed a crime. He agreed but said that he didn't know what he was anxious about.

Commentary

In this session, he is again preoccupied with his inner persecutory objects and mainly I am not in his mind at all. There are two occasions in the session when he does, however, notice me. One occasion he thinks that I am complaining about him when I mention that he has been in this position before; that is, he sees me as impatient and critical. When I describe this to him, however, it doesn't alleviate the anxiety. The outer objects in his life (including me) are infused with the persecutory feeling and when I describe his view of me as negative and judgemental, he agrees with this, and doesn't acknowledge that this might be his perception rather than the reality. (Incidentally I wasn't aware of feeling judgemental or critical about him in this session, although it was important to think about whether I might have been in supervision.) Again, I don't directly address his delusional belief, but I do suggest that it might be motivated as an explanation of his anxious mood. As he is not certain that his beliefs are true, this suggestion makes sense to him in a way that it wouldn't if he were absolutely certain that it was true and didn't believe that he had an emotional problem and is a hypothetical reformulation of his current situation.

Later Session

He had got angry at home and smashed things up. He had gone to the emergency department. He stayed a little while but left before being seen. A friend he met in the mental health service decided to stop being his friend. He worries that he might have said something about defrauding social security to his ex-friend and that now he will take revenge on him by informing on him. He has been trying to remember if he had spoken to him about this. He had had a fight with his father. He felt that his father was being unreasonable. His father wouldn't stop complaining. Tom got tense and felt like hurting someone or himself so instead he smashed up the room. I asked him what, with hindsight he felt he should have done and he said he should have walked away. In this session, the persecuting object is located not in the government but in his ex-friend who has cut him off and who he now fears may take revenge on him for not approving of his texts, and then in his father who keeps making unreasonable demands on him. He complains about his father complaining, but of course in the session, it is the client who is complaining to the therapist.

A Later Session

There had been a phone call to the ward and he had answered it. It had been a father wanting to speak to his son, and he had confused Tom with his son. He hates being confused with other people. He had been talking to some of his friends when on leave and he worried that he might have said some things that were anti-feminist and that this might get back to a friend who would be offended. But he wasn't sure if he had said these things or not. I said that his doubt about his memory was linked to his self-esteem. He agreed and said that he thought his paranoia wasn't just about his brain but was about his feelings. After a pause, he said that medication did help a lot. He asked me if he was talking rubbish. I said that he felt he wasn't doing the therapy right, and that this was another example of his self-doubt. He said that the DBT session had been about acceptance and he had not liked it. He said it would be good if he could accept what his parents had done but he couldn't. He keeps remembering being hurt, and he gets angry and then has temper outbursts. He thinks that his parents are not well, why is it him that has to get drugged, not them? And then he had watched a programme about people with heart failure and he had become very emotional. He said that he feels sad about his father (who was in heart failure) as well as hating him and he doesn't get it. I said that he had mixed feelings. He said that he would have liked a different father, and in his family there hadn't been any physical affection. He then brought up a fight he had had with his girlfriend over her weight, and at the end they had resolved it. I said that this was a different end to that with his father.

Commentary

In this session, the theme of his relationship to his father, rather than delusional persecution, runs through this session. He was disturbed by a father who confuses his son with Tom. One way in which this is disturbing is that he has a fragile hold of his own identity and other people confusing his identity adds to this anxiety. He is concerned about whether he is using our sessions well, and this is a doubt as to whether our connection is being helpful and, as I am a father figure in the transference, this is again an anxiety about connection to a father. He then goes on to talk about acceptance as a goal which he has heard about in DBT. He cannot forgive his father but realises that he also wants a father's love. He wishes he had had a different father (which takes us back to the beginning of the session, but also suggests that he might hope to find another father in the therapist). He is less preoccupied with his delusional ideas here and more with the problem of feeling unloved by his father, which is progress. It seems to him that acceptance in his situation would be to accept that his treatment by his parents was ok and that he has to accept being haunted by bad objects from his past. He feels that acceptance would mean his feelings about his father were invalid. He tries to use assertiveness strategies towards his family but he just doesn't want to use these strategies. The problem for him is that he doesn't feel independent of his parents. He not only hates them but also needs them. So, he is stuck. In Fairbairn's language, he hasn't achieved mature dependence but is relying on parents who have not met his needs. So, he can't win. And to accept this situation seems to him to be accepting the unacceptable. However, that he is talking about these issues in therapy, rather than being preoccupied with his paranoid fears, is obviously a sign that he is much improved.

Later Session

We had to use a different room and he mentioned that it had a strange smell. He had had a fight with a friend over having someone trans-gender at a party. He got really angry with her. He then went on to tell me that his medication had been changed, so as he is calmer and he just said what he thought and isn't worried about it. He is not so worried about Tony Blair or messages from the TV. He still gets these thoughts but isn't bothered by them. He said that he is going to be signed off as sick and won't need to look for work. He has mixed feelings about this. He doesn't have to worry about finding a job, but he feels insulted. He said that he had gone out with his partner's father who had bought him lunch. He didn't want to eat as he is in a reducing phase of his bodybuilding. I said that I thought the focus on his body was linked to being unhappy. He took this on board and said he was unhappy about everything in his life and began to weep. He talked about various ways he could kill himself. I reflected that he was feeling hopeless and he said that everything goes wrong and that he thinks it will never get better. He stopped himself crying and I said that he didn't feel comfortable getting sad in our session and he agreed and said that he thought I might laugh at him. I said that he felt I felt superior to him. He then told me of a dream in which his psychiatrist was looking after a horse. He tried to get the attention of his psychiatrist but he kept brushing the horse. I commented that in the dream the psychiatrist was too busy looking after the horse to bother with him. He said that he had been reading about people with bi-polar and they list all these celebrities with bi-polar. But he can't do anything, so how come? Or are they lying about the celebrities really having bi-polar?

Commentary on the Session

In this session, the delusional ideas have faded to thoughts that he doesn't believe in and isn't preoccupied with, although they still come into his head. When I link his preoccupation with his weight to his unhappiness, he doesn't bat this away, as he had in previous sessions, but picks it up and elaborates it, in that he says he feels unhappy about everything in his life and that nothing ever works out. But he stops himself crying about this because of the fear that I will humiliate him and he continues this theme by telling me of a dream in which his psychiatrist is obsessed with his own interests and is uninterested in helping him, which I took as a picture of his perception of his relationship with me. This not only relates to his idea that I will laugh at him but also links back to his memories of his father as coldly critical and despising. When he was delusional he felt he was going to be found out for having committed all the crimes that he heard of and that he would be punished for these crimes. He had felt that he was being conspired against by an external force, maybe the Prime Minister. Now that he is no longer psychotic he fears that life will let him down and that I look down on him and will treat him with contempt and will humiliate him if he shows me his sadness. The theme is the same. That he brings this up in the therapy with me is a sign that the rapport between us has increased.

A Later Session

He arrived early and looked bright.

He said that the new medication really worked. He went to visit his part-ners' family and the TV was on and it had been a long time before he had realised that the programme was about the police. That hadn't happened in two years. He had been using a desensitisation method which he thought (mistakenly) I had suggested-thinking about the police when relaxed- and that had worked too. He isn't feeling anxious all the time. His parents are selling the house and this worried him. There had been an open house and there had been children in his room. He worried that one of the kids could have picked up some of his notes about the police. He is more able to use the DBT skills when calm he said. A woman in the skills group (who was also a client of mine) said that, at the end of the programme, she wouldn't be able to see her therapist any more. He had wondered what would hap-pen when he finished DBT. I said that he might miss seeing me. He said he didn't like that way of talking about it as it made him sound dependent. He said that if he had to have a different therapist it would take a couple of weeks to get used to them as he had been used to talking to me. He finds it hard to use IE skills with his parents because he doesn't really respect them. I said that he had some reason to feel aggrieved with them but that feel-ing that and acting on it weren't the same thing. He noticed that he can be rejecting of being touched by his girlfriend.

Commentary on the Session

The session begins with optimism. The new medication has made a dra-matic, positive difference to his state of mind, and this is very encouraging for him. He has also been trying the cognitive therapy techniques he is learning in the DBT group and is finding that they help. Even when he returns home to find his bedroom occupied by children and worries about them having taken his notes about the police, his worries are not that he has committed a terrible crime, but that his notes on having committed a terrible crime will be misunderstood, and he can dismiss these thoughts.

He then brings three problems. (1) How to use his DBT skills with his parents when he doesn't feel like being respectful? (2) He has been feeling rejecting of his partner and gets irritated with her if she shows affection. (3) He has a worry about what will happen to his relationship with me at the end of DBT. These are all linked. He is pointing out that the assertiveness strategies aren't going to change his resentment towards his parents. His feelings towards his parents are reflected in how he finds himself reacting to his partner. He expresses a worry about whether the individual therapy will end when the skills group ends. I suggest to him that he is might find it difficult if the therapy were to end and he denies this, and doesn't want to hear about being dependant on me in any way. For him, the idea of depending on someone fills him with anxiety, as he fears that this will leave him vulnerable to being hurt. So, the same feeling comes up with his parents, his current partner and in the therapy, and it is not difficult to link it to its origins in his childhood. He resists this suggestion. There is no talk of the paranoid ideas, apart from reflection on techniques to stop thinking about them, which already implies that he regards them as an unpleasant symptom to be dealt with rather than a danger to be pondered on. He is stuck in depending on people who he feels he can't manage without and yet are bad. So, for example, he feels that he is improving and then worries that seeing me will get taken away from him. But he can't acknowledge this because to depend on someone makes him vulnerable to being hurt.

A Later Session

He hadn't come to a session for three weeks. He had told the psychiatrist that I was working with the government. He began by saying that everything was a mess. He had been hearing voices telling him to confess to planting a bomb. He has two memories, that he made a bomb and that he didn't and doesn't know which is the right one. He thinks though that it can't be right as he doesn't know how to make a bomb. But the voices keep telling him to confess and he isn't sure which memory is right. And he broke up with Tracey. He thought that the relationship hadn't been right for a long time. I said that this had been a sudden change and that he had previously felt good about having been in a stable relationship. He ignored this and went on that now he is worried that she will get revenge on him. The voice was saying that she was behind him on the street. He worries that she will tell people private things about him. If she does, however, he can retaliate. I said he now felt that his partner, who he had found supportive, was now someone he felt he had to protect himself from. He said that he felt guilty all the time. He apologised for saying that I was working with the government. I said he felt I couldn't be trusted and that I thought that the closer he got to people the more vulnerable he felt and the more he felt he was in danger. He said that he had thought there was a camera in the room with me. He said that he hadn't been coming, because he felt that I was working against him with the government.

Commentary on the Session

This was the first session after three missed appointments. In previous sessions, he has been talking about how he was finding that he was getting irritated with his girlfriend and that he didn't like to be touched by her. In this session, he is feeling persecuted on all sides. He has recurred to the state of mind he was in previously. Voices are telling him that he should confess to planting a bomb, and he has memories of planting the bomb and not planting the bomb. He cannot distinguish between his memory and a fear or fantasy of him doing something criminal. He had the intuition that I was spying on him, and believed this so that he didn't come to his appointment. He thought I was feeling vengeful towards him and the voices tell him that his girlfriend is going to get revenge on him, possibly by telling people embarrassing things about him. He takes this seriously enough that he has prepared a response–which is that he will take counter-revenge on her. And he is back to worrying about crimes he may have committed. He has returned to feeling that he is surrounded by people who want to harm him, and the delusional ideas about having committed a serious crime are back. The delusional ideas seem part of his general feeling that relationships are too dangerous for him. Now he fears that he will be punished for bailing out—and he bailed out because he was scared of getting trapped. Obviously in this situation, the most useful thing is to respond to the general problem that he is having and that isn't going to be coping with the psychotic experiences as if they were unrelated to his general situation. It is important that he has returned to therapy to talk about his problems and wants to apologise to me for having thought I was plotting against him. He ended his relationship quite precipitously, and this is an example of splitting. The object is either good or bad, and having become bad must be got rid of. I talked to him about things changing suddenly, but he doesn't really pick up on what I am talking about, presumably because from his position it seems unrelated to what he is concerned about.

A Later Session

He said that he was feeling depressed. He had been having some physical symptoms and saw a doctor who thought it could be a physical illness and has sent him for tests. The psychiatrist had said it was an anxiety symptom.

He is worried about being ill and also worried about not being ill and it being in his mind. I said that he couldn't win either way. He said the physical symptoms didn't occur when he was anxious so he has been worried about being ill. He pointed out that this was strange, as only a couple of weeks ago he had wanted to die. I said that he felt as if there was someone around waiting to blame him for not being physically ill. He said that he liked the medication that he is on, as although he has no motivation, he has better control of his anxiety and is less impulsive. He doesn't take overdoses like he did. Recently though he was tempted to take an overdose, having come across a couple of old boxes of medication. He hadn't done it because he didn't want to go back to hospital. Some nurses are really nasty people. He has been panicking about whether he filled out the social security forms incorrectly. He pointed out it was time to finish.

General Commentary

At times, Tom presents his problem as being persecuted by the government or having been responsible for various crimes. The evidence for this is often a fantasy that he confuses with a memory. At other times, it is an idea of reference, and at other times, it is just a strong intuition. He moves in and out of the delusion. This occurs against a background of feelings and ideas which are not delusional but which are, nevertheless, persecutory. His idea that he is being spied on by the government is delusional. The idea that his ex-girlfriend will take revenge on him isn't delusional and, of course could turn out to be true, but is persecutory. When he moves out of home and begins to worry that his flatmates are going to turn against him, this sounds like anxiety, but with a persecutory theme. The point is that his life problems and his delusional symptom are really all of a kind. Tom was delusional for six months, but was already in therapy before this. I was working with him on his anxiety and self-esteem and then his self-harm. Once he became delusional I worked with him on elaborating the context in which these ideas had occurred and increasing his understanding of that process rather than directly challenging the belief. When I raise the idea that he might worry about me disappearing, he is quick to let me know that this isn't about me, because he wouldn't find it acceptable to depend on me, but is about being supported. The theme that runs through these sessions in both psychotic and non-psychotic forms is the conflict of wanting to be loved and fearing that being close to someone will make him vulnerable to being hurt. This theme is a repetition of his experiences with his parents in his childhood and his teenage years in particular. This comes up in the therapy, as he not only continues to come and at times share painful feelings but also wants to avoid it. Here the idea of the therapist being personally important to him is threatening and he turns a blind eye to this, presumably because of these difficult experiences of being dependant on his parents. It would really have been good to be able to go on seeing him for several further years.

With Tom, because he has relationships and has not withdrawn completely into his inner world, it is possible to discuss this theme and the idea that he might have fears about his relationship to me, and that his delusional ideas of persecution might relate to his disappointments in his parents.

June

June was a 32-year-old woman whom I saw in the Psychotherapy Department in Hackney. She had numerous admissions after taking overdoses, but she had also heard voices about which she had fluctuating insight. She lived with her daughter in a council flat in a high-rise block in Tower Hamlets. She had had several admissions mainly due to parasuicide acts, in which she had been quite thought disordered and had had command hallucinations. The psychiatrists were not sure of her diagnosis, but she was referred due to her frequent admissions to hospital. I saw her as part of the DBT programme. I had been working with her for six months during which time she had few suicidal feelings or voices, and we had mainly worked on her positive goals. However, at this half way point in the therapy she became depressed and this seemed to be out of the blue. She began to hear the voices again telling her that she was bad and should harm herself. She could not identify any problem that seemed to be the cause of her low mood. She had begun a casual job which had not worked out and I wondered if this had been the trigger. A functional analysis of exacerbations of her low mood had not really led to any clear internal or external triggers. She had negative thoughts about not having much money and negative thoughts about her appearance and her character. She thought that her life would not improve, that she would never hold down a job and that she would always be on her own.

After three months of feeling depressed, June came to a session and said that she had had feelings of suicidality at the weekend and had heard voices telling her to kill herself. I asked her what her been going on but she couldn't think of any obvious stresses at that time. However, in the previous session, she had mentioned incidentally that it was only two weeks until the court case against her ex-partner began and I pointed this out. I had known that there was to be a trial against him, but I had not known exactly when this was to be. She said that she kept forgetting that it was going to happen soon, and then remembering. I suggested that she kept forgetting that it was about to happen as a way of avoiding the painful feelings about the trial, and the events that had happened in her past. Her ex-partner, who she had been separated from for two years, had seriously assaulted her and he was being prosecuted for this assault. She had been having thoughts about her life being hopeless and there being no point going on. We did a role play around this, using an empty chair in which we imagined the voice being in the chair. In the chair, being her negative voice, she told herself that there was no point going on, that she was worthless and that nothing would get any better for her. Back in the other chair she struggled to talk back to counter the voice. She told the voice that things didn't have to be hopeless, but wasn't very convincing. June found some relief from this, but she said that she still felt that some of what the voices said was true (so that she wasn't going with the idea of thinking of herself in different parts). She told me that in the previous year she had spent most of the time believing that her mother was poisoning her with the medication that she gave her (the prescribed psychiatric medication that is), and hearing voices telling her to harm herself. The anti-psychotic medication had, however, reduced the frequency of the voices. I asked her how she felt about this. She said that in some ways it had been easier when she heard negative voices rather than having negative thoughts. And when she believed that her mother was poisoning her, this was easier than how things were now. (I didn't suggest this to her, she suggested it herself.) What she was saying was that her psychotic symptoms (delusions and auditory hallucinations) reduced her level of anxiety by projecting the dangers out into the environment. It was easier to struggle with a voice that wants to harm you rather than with a thought that you want to harm yourself. Later on in therapy she told me that she realised that the voices came more when she was listening for them. If she avoided doing this, the voices did not come.

After a while, she liked role playing assertive responses to her voices using the empty chair technique. This was teaching a coping skill for dealing with her voices and for dealing with her self-attacks, because the inner critic and the voices were saying very similar things. However, it was also role playing someone standing up for her in a way that she hadn't had from her parents. Her father had left her when she was very young. Her mother had struggled with her own psychological problems and had not been emotionally available and when she was being bullied at school she felt that no one was looking out for her. Now I think most importantly this wasn't just a role play of someone looking out for her. It was the fact that I was actually looking out for her, so that that she experienced me as supportive and as a "good object" that was helpful.

It can be argued that such voices as these are a different phenomenon to those of clients with "schizophrenia" and a number of attempts have been made to set up criteria for this; for example, Schneider suggested that voices in the third person were indications that the person had schizophrenia; others have suggested that where the voice seems to be located can be used as a criterion. However, none of these criteria seem to differentiate the voices of schizophrenia from the voices of personality disorder (Slotema et al., 2012).

Reference

Slotema, C. W., Daalman, K., Blom, J. D., Diederen, K. M., Hoek, H. W., & Sommer, I. E. (2012). Auditory verbal hallucinations in patients with borderline personality disorder are similar to those in schizophrenia. *Psychological Medicine*, 2(9), 1873–1878.

10 Jean

The Girl Who Never Left Home—A General Failure to Thrive

Jean was referred to the psychotherapy department of the Dartford Mental Health Trust by her Consultant Psychiatrist. She had grown up in Dartford, East London. She presented with persecutory auditory hallucinations, persecutory delusions, and negative symptoms. She also was chronically depressed. She had difficulties with self-care; sometimes she was smelly or had food on her clothes. She withdrew from social contact to a large degree. She had the experience/belief that others could read her mind. She had been seen in the mental health service for over 20 years. She had command hallucinations which ordered her to kill herself, and auditory hallucinations that put her down and threatened her. She was referred to me for help with her voices. She would periodically get admitted to hospital following a suicidal act, or with plans to kill herself. The voices told her that she should die or that she was worthless. Sometimes she would step out in front of a car in response to her persecutory voices.

She saw me for a year during which I worked with her on strategies to cope with the voices, and plans to avoid self-harm. After this she saw another psychologist. She told her that she had been sexually abused as a child. And, when she left the service, the psychologist referred her back to me to deal with this issue. I saw her on a weekly or fortnightly basis for several years.

I first met Jean when she was around 45 years of age. Her psychiatrist hoped that psychological therapy could help her to cope with her voices. She was diagnosed with treatment-resistant schizophrenia. She lived with her daughter. She had a part time job as a cleaner. She was a tall, overweight woman who had a somewhat defeated air. She never smiled. She did indeed hear voices that put her down and threatened her. They also told her to kill herself. Her mood was chronically low and she would periodically get admitted to hospital. Once she was in hospital, she often spent long periods there as she would say that she would like to die and had thoughts and plans to kill herself. And these chronic suicidal ideas didn't pass.

She had been living with her daughter since her husband had left her 5 years ago. She was involved with a number of mental health service activities; for example, she was part of a committee which looked at the

DOI:10.4324/9781003168379-12

consumer's view of what the mental health service provided. She had one sister who was married and who had a child. She lived in another city about 100 miles away. One of the first things that was noticeable about her was that she often left the session about 20 minutes early (that is after about half an hour). However, she came to almost all her appointments when she was not detained in hospital.

When I began to see her for the second time, she was still bothered by voices, but she began to tell me about other symptoms that she had. In her first session with me (after she had been re-referred), I mentioned that she had said that she wanted to work on the sexual abuse she had been subjected to as a child. She acknowledged this but didn't elaborate on this at the time, however.

She found it difficult to take care of herself and her home and she had carers that cleaned the house for her. She was obese and had other physical problems that made it difficult for her to shop and clean, in addition to her lack of motivation. She felt guilty, and she believed that she was going to be punished for her perceived sins. She had withdrawn from people and saw almost no one except for mental health workers and her daughter.

She had visual hallucinations of groups of men in her house. She thought that these men were neo-Nazis who appeared to her in order to torment her. She was very fearful that they would harm her or assault her. She thought that the voices she heard were the voices of the person who abused her and the neo-Nazis. Sometimes she would be trapped in her flat, because she was too frightened to go past these men. Because she felt that people could read her mind she avoided travelling on public transport as much as she could. She had olfactory hallucinations of sulphur. One strategy she had developed to deal with this experience was to self-harm. This seemed to both be a distraction, an unconscious form of self-punishment, and be a placation of the voice telling her to kill herself. Her abuser was at the head of the conspiracy of neo-Nazis who wanted to harm her, or sexually assault her. At other times, she would act on the voices telling her to kill herself and make an impulsive suicidal gesture.

She told me that she had been sexually abused by her cousin when she was very young and this had continued into her 20s, even after she was married and she felt very ashamed of it. She hadn't been able to talk about this with her parents who had been too busy arguing. Eventually her father left home when she was 10 and she never saw him again. She had got married in her late teens. She had a daughter and, when her daughter was in primary school, she had had an affair and left home. After a few months she returned to her husband. He took her back but after this always treated her with contempt and would often bring up her affair in front of her children. She saw her sister once a year when she went to stay with her over Christmas.

When her psychosis had first begun, she had been working on the till in a supermarket. She said that she began to experience her thoughts leaving her head and affecting things in the world. So, if she thought about something it would happen. She could affect people's reactions. Later she said that she would notice references to her in various places. For example, she saw a news stand and she thought that this referred to her because "News" rhymes with "Jews" and she had some Jewish ancestry. She didn't have a clear account of how the incident with the news stand could have happened. She believed that, at that time, when it all began, she had developed special, paranormal powers. She had had the idea that there were a group of gangsters who wanted her to help them with her special powers. Some of the people that came into the supermarket looked suspicious and she thought they were gangsters. She thought they wanted to abduct her and get her to use her paranormal powers to commit crime. By the time she met me, she no longer experienced these paranormal powers.

In the present, she no longer thought she was conspired against by gangsters but thought that she was being conspired against by a group of neo-Nazis. If she saw someone of a middle-eastern appearance at the bus stop, she thought that they were there to spy on her.

The first stage of therapy with Jean consisted of developing coping skills to cope with her auditory hallucinations and feelings of paranoia. I gave her a list of different strategies that people used to cope with their voices and asked her what she did to cope. She could sometimes distract herself from the voices. She found music or TV were helpful, particularly as she had very little contact with people. If she did what the voice told her (self- harming) the voices would let up. I tried role playing a dialogue with the voice. We talked to the voice imagined as sitting in an empty chair and asked the voice what it was doing and why. The voice being Hitler turned out to be motivated by pure malice. It wanted to harm her to cause her pain. We worked on trying to tell the voice to stop trying to harm her, but the voice was not affected by these protestations. If she cut herself, the voices stopped. But trying to stand up to the voice or banish it did not help her. Maybe this partly depends on the client's perception of the identity of the voice. I suggested that we set up a challenge to the power of the voice by suggesting that the voice might harm me. Jean was not persuaded of the relevance of this. It wasn't that she argued against this as a test of the truth of the idea that the voice (Hitler) was all powerful it was, I think, that I hadn't been able to induce her to take seriously the hypothesis that she might be mistaken about this. The voice was Hitler and self-evidently evil and powerful.

Following this, I decided to try to work on her belief in her delusion. I put it to Jean that her belief that there was a conspiracy was one explanation of her experiences, but that it was also possible that the voices and feelings of people conspiring against her were symptoms of her depression (she acknowledged that she was depressed although she wasn't convinced that she had psychotic disorder). She clearly didn't think that this was a useful line of enquiry.

I talked with her about her belief that her father was one of the voices that came to torment her. This seemed inconsistent with her belief that her father was dead. Of course, it would be possible to hold both of these beliefs consistently by claiming that the voice was of her father's ghost or spirit, but she didn't say this. She believed that her father was dead and that her father was alive and the inconsistence between these statements didn't really influence her. One could suggest that this was a feature of the state of mind she was in. That she was able to hold inconsistent beliefs was a regressed state of thinking, (although this could be true, it is also true that holding on to emotionally important beliefs in the face of evidence that they are false is a rather common experience.)

Jean's attitude to coming was very interesting. Although my attempts to enhance her coping skills to empower her in her relationship with the voices, or to challenge the truth of her delusion, were all really a failure she continued to come regularly. She very rarely missed a session. However, she also never stayed for more than 30 minutes. She had an approach-avoidant attitude to the therapy. Sometimes it would be clear that voices were talking to her and this was often voices telling her to leave or that she couldn't trust me. Other times she would leave as she found the session exhausting.

Jean's conscious motivation to come to the sessions was, I think, to talk about having been abused rather than to get help with her voices, and this is why she continued to come, but couldn't stay. This expressed her attitude to talking about what had happened to her.

Conceptualising Jean using a cognitive therapy lens, we can say that she has a delusional belief that she is being persecuted by Hitler, the disciples of Hitler, her cousin, and her father. They are conspiring to harm her, to kill her or rape her. This delusion is based on hearing voices that tell her that this is so. How this belief began is really lost in the mists of time as she has had this belief for over 20 years. She has a relationship with the voices of subjugated victim to powerful abuser. This relationship is similar to that that she had with her cousin who abused her and her father who eventually abandoned her. Her pervasively low mood probably contributes to her low self-esteem and makes it hard to take any action to get out of the situation that she is in. She experiences having her mind read and this also adds to her idea that she is being persecuted, although it is unclear why she hears voices or why she believes that the voices are real. It is clear that there is some relationship in this case with her childhood experiences but, of course, although she was certainly treated badly and abused, no one threatened to kill her and there were some positive times with her parents, unlike with Hitler. These experiences are clearly not memories but may be transformed memories.

Thinking psychodynamically, Jean's problems can be seen in the following light. Jean has retreated from relationships with other people, not only in the external world but also psychologically. When she leaves home, she is terrified by intrusions into her mind from others. Her social world has shrunk and she largely lives in a world peopled by her persecutory objects which are projected into the environment as persecutory voices and visions of persecutory people. She has little contact with others and this leaves her with her internal objects. Her sense of hopelessness comes from this. There is no getting away from her abusive cousin and the dead abandoning father who is also not dead. She describes a horribly traumatic childhood.

Thinking about Jean's problems in this way helps in a number of ways. First, it explains why she might persist in coming to therapy when the strategies I had used with her had clearly not been successful. Her life had been a retreat from an early trauma and loss. Her cousin had abused her and her father abandoned her and Jean's marriage ended up as a repeat of the relationship with her father. At one point, she told me, she had told her mother about the sexual abuse, and her mother had reacted by ignoring what she said and leaving the room. In the relationship with the therapist, a part of Jean wants to find an alternative to her parent's version of love.

Fairbairn's (1952) suggestion that the neglected or abused child blames himself or herself in order to preserve the abusive parent as good, because the child cannot survive without the parent, may explain Jean's conviction that she was responsible for having been abused and not protected by her parents. Why in her case the trauma results in a psychosis rather than a neurotic or borderline presentation is important, but unknown.

In the sessions with me, her understanding was that she would benefit from talking about what had happened to her as a child. She would begin to talk about this sometimes but the voices would threaten her and she would have to stop. Furthermore, she did not relax into talking in the sessions. She always seemed wary even before the voices began to threaten her in the middle of the session. Why was this? I thought that she had a conflict between an inner child part of her which wanted to be able to grieve about her childhood and be comforted, and an inner critic who just wanted to punish her for what she had done.

I found myself liking Jean. At times I also found myself seriously concerned about her welfare, particularly when she was cutting herself or feeling like jumping in front of a car. However, I also felt that I didn't really have a client in therapy. Although I booked her in for hour long appointments after a short time, I realised that she wouldn't stay for the full session. From her point of view, she is wanting to talk about being abused by her cousin. From my point of view she is in conflict about whether to talk about what had happened to her. One part of her doesn't want to talk about it and this part is projected out into the voices which attack her for wanting to talk. This can be thought of as her inner abusive object who threatens her for wanting to talk. So, thought of this way, it is an enactment of an interpersonal situation she was in countless times as a young woman. Her leaving the session after 30 minutes made it hard to develop a conversation with her about any of this.

Thinking of her leaving early as motivated by being unable to talk about the trauma, made it easier for me not to act out in the counter-transference by becoming annoyed with her for just dipping her toe into the sessions, but then exiting. After all, as well as her own shame and feelings of responsibility for what had happened, she had also been ignored by her mother when she had told her about it.

She saw me as a benign person in her life. Her relationship to her mother in her early childhood may be the model for this positive relationship in her life. However, I was up against Hitler and found wanting in dealing with her persecutors. In this, I thought, there was a repetition of her relationship with her mother, who was a benign figure, but powerless to deal with her cousin or father.

During the height of her psychosis, she experienced her thoughts and feelings in a concrete way. Thinking or feeling something was able to harm someone.

The positive part of the therapy was that she persisted in attending the sessions, even though she still had to leave the sessions under threat. In her case, she really waited for me to direct the conversation. There is the beginning of a positive relationship between the client and me but it is threatened by the destructive actions of a bad object, perceived as an abusive, bullying voice. The problem is what to do about the abbreviation of sessions. Obviously with a non-psychotic client, the therapist would bring up the repeated leaving early and wonder if it was, for example, motivated by ambivalence. But in the present situation, as the client's perception is that it is an external voice, this will make no sense. She feels that she is leaving, because she is under threat from an external voice. So, the comment would seem to make no sense.

Reference

Fairbairn, C. (1952). *Psychoanalytic studies of the personality*. London: Routledge.

11 Steven

The Gangster's Ex-Boyfriend— A Repetition of Abuse 2

I first met Steven on an inpatient unit in Campbelltown in Sydney. He had been admitted due to an emotional crisis and had taken an overdose. I was introduced to him during a ward round. The psychiatrist asked him to see me to help him with his delusions and he gave me a suspicious look, as he didn't believe that he had any delusions to be helped with. He had been in hospital for a couple of weeks. He had been having thoughts of killing himself. He heard voices telling him to kill himself much of the time.

He was 31 years old and he lived in a mental health hostel. He had no contact with his family had no friends and was supported by various mental health workers. He was slightly underweight and had a troubled demeanour. He did not work and hadn't had a full-time job for many years. He had great difficult shopping due to pervasive anxiety and attacks of panic. This anxiety was not about having a panic attack or having a heart attack or having an illness or being judged; he was worried about being attacked. He had a number of different diagnoses. Some people thought that he had borderline personality disorder; others thought that he could have schizophrenia or schizoaffective disorder. He did really present symptoms from all of these categories. I began to see him as an outpatient and I continued to see him for the best part of five years.

He had had a very difficult life. He had been brought up by his parents in a suburb of Sydney. He was the middle child of three. He took some time to explain his story to me. His parents were unhappily married and he remembered them fighting most of the time when he was a child. He was severely neglected. He remembers going to school smelly and being teased by the other children because of this. An indication of the degree of neglect is that Steven and his brothers were often not fed. He wasn't able to concentrate at school due to the situation at home and because he had become a pariah at school. Going to school was another experience of defeat and he became mildly delinquent. He was sexually abused by an uncle when he was ten and his parents broke up when he was 12. After his mother threw his father out, his father descended into heroin addiction and he remembers feeling sorry for him. Shortly after his parents separated, his mother moved his (Steven's) step-father into the house. His stepfather argued with Steven's father. When

DOI:10.4324/9781003168379-13

Steven's father hit Steven his step-father beat him up. However, he didn't feel protected by this. Rather he felt to blame for his father being hurt. He also felt to blame for having been beaten. In addition to the neglect, abuse, and public humiliation that he suffered, there was no positive person in his story. All the men in his life seemed to harm him in one way or another. He didn't really describe his mother as being involved in his life at all. He didn't have a relative or school teacher to mitigate the unrelenting misery of his family life.

In his mid-teens as the house was overcrowded, he moved out and got a job in a factory. He rented a room as a lodger in a house. He saw his mother occasionally, but didn't really feel welcome when he went home. He felt anxious around other people and didn't go out to socialise very often. When he did it would be with other workers in the factory. After a year, he began a relationship and moved in with an older man, Tom. Tom had a history of violence, however, and became jealous and suspicious and began to beat him. Tom had a criminal record for violence in the past, which attracted Steven to him as he felt he would defend him from the dangers in the world. Unfortunately, he needed defending from him. So, he found himself back in a similar position to that he had been in his childhood. In his mid-20s, Steven left him and it was at this point that he developed a paranoid belief and began to hear voices. He had been living in housing provided by the mental health service since that time.

When I first saw him, he was anxious but didn't seem particularly suspicious of me. Over the next few weeks, he began to explain his story. His main problems as he saw them were that he was being conspired against by a group of terrorists who wanted to harm him. He feared being raped or murdered. He had no doubts about this belief. At times of stress, he was more preoccupied with this belief, but he was always worried about it. Current evidence he had for the belief was that he saw a group of men wearing hoodies in his garden at night. He would peer out through the window of his flat and would see them at the bottom of the garden. He rated his degree of conviction in this being a group of men conspiring to hurt him at 100% or Absolutely Certain.

In addition, he had periods when he would believe that he was a different person with a different name and go off looking for where he lived. He told me that he remembered little of these experiences or what he did. This seems to be a dissociative phenomenon. It occurred when he was going through periods of extreme stress. He also heard voices which threatened him and told him to cut himself or kill himself and he felt that these voices related to the men that were waiting at bottom of his garden. He thought other people could read his mind and spied on his movements. Occasionally he received letters or notes left in his room that he believed came from the people who were trying to harm him. The idea that these notes were written by him didn't seem possible to him. He had, then, a longstanding delusional belief, voices, and visions which confirmed the belief and periods of fugue which he mainly didn't relate to the conspiracy (the exception being the notes written by someone else). His belief that the Satan worshipers were gaining access to his room was very disturbing to him.

After he had got a little used to being with me, we began to work on modifying his delusional belief. The belief dominated much of his life so I began with trying to modify the delusion. He agreed to try this out and we began by looking for an alternative explanation for his experiences. (In this case, one does not have to look very far to see the connections between his psychotic symptoms and his developmental history. He, of course, did not see this. Although the experiences seem to be rooted in his experience of trauma and abuse this didn't seem to be the place to start.) I set up the alternative hypothesis that these experiences (hearing voices, seeing hooded men in the garden, finding notes in his room) were linked to being depressed. Looking at alternative explanations for the evidence (e.g. that seeing the group of men at the bottom of the garden was an expression of his fear of being hurt) did not get very far so we moved on to setting up a behavioural test of his belief.

One piece of evidence that confirmed his delusion was his belief that people stared at him in the street. He thought that they did this because they could read his thoughts. And this was part of a conspiracy to monitor and harm him. I suggested that we go out into the street together as a behavioural experiment and to observe whether other people were looking at him or not. My role here was to be truthful about whether I could see people looking at him. I was a method of testing his perceptions of the situation. As we walked down the street what I mainly noticed was that he kept looking over his shoulder, looking very tense and very obvious. Later we discussed whether he had felt people were looking at him and that I hadn't noticed anyone looking at him. I suggested that when he looked around to see if anyone was looking at him this might attract attention. His degree of belief in his delusions did indeed decrease to some degree.

I carried on seeing him once we had completed the challenging of his delusional belief. There had been some moderate amount of change. But his life was not really any better. He moved into a different hostel and there one of his support workers told him that he believed that there was a conspiracy to commit terrorism going on and confirmed Steven's delusional belief. This was unfortunate, to say the least.

Steven had a series of traumatic experiences during his childhood and this, together with the absence of a supportive figure, set up a persecutory inner object and a reciprocal victimised inner child. His father was not only a persecuting figure but also a damaged figure throughout his childhood. Of course, he needed his love but ended up with him abandoning him and making him feel like a despised object rather than a person. His mother on the other hand was an absent neglecting figure who didn't provide care for her children. It is difficult for him to care for himself and organise his life when he is identified with a neglecting, absent mother.

His self-harm and suicidality are attacks on him by his inner abandoning father, or abusive uncle, or neglecting mother. The dilemma for him as a child was that the only attention, he received was abusive attention. His relationships outside of the family seem to repetitions of his abusive childhood experiences, for example with his ex-boyfriend. His boyfriend becomes an external persecutory object, and this becomes another traumatic experience, and a repetition. His boyfriend acts out the persecution with him; he has projected his inner abusive/abandoning object into his ex-partner and the scene re-enacts his inner emotional world. He hallucinated what he expects to find. In his sessions with me, he didn't bring other problems to the session. He talked about his fears about what might harm him, and reported on his other symptoms but didn't bring personal things to the session.

When psychological therapy allows space for the client to bring things along to talk about and the client doesn't, this is obviously a move in the relationship between the client and the therapist that may have a meaning. Of course, he didn't have very much going on in his current life, he had no friends, wasn't in touch with his family and didn't work, but he could have talked about the past or his hopes for the future. He had told me his life history, of course, but that was a part of taking a personal history. In addition, he didn't elaborate on his feelings. The effect of not bringing things to talk about was that I took the lead in asking things about what had been happening. This felt to me that he was not engaging with aspects of his life. Also, that one effect of focusing on his delusional beliefs was to avoid strong emotions about some of the traumatic events in his life. In keeping his distance from these thoughts and feelings, he was also, of course, keeping his distance from me. The lack of depth of his relationship with me mirrored his own avoidance of his own feelings. The feelings of fear and anger are directed at the delusional persecutors. He avoids these feelings in respect of the people that they really belong to. What is the therapist to do? One approach is to use imagery or the empty chair technique to evoke feelings about the figures from the past. One could ask him to imagine his interactions with his parents or the teacher or his ex-partner. The nearest I got to this was when he described in detail the way his uncle abused him. Actually, describing in detail what happened to him was really quite powerful, but as it was me that had suggested this to him, he remained a passive avoider in relation to memories of traumas of the past.

12 Theresa

The Drive to Succeed— Delusion and Recovery

Theresa had a diagnosis of schizoaffective disorder or schizophrenia. She was referred to the Psychotherapy Department of the City and Hackney Mental Health Trust. At that time, the psychotherapy service was located in a house just outside the Homerton Hospital on a residential street. She was 28 and had recently been discharged from hospital after trying to kill herself. She had made a noose and had gone into the garage and hung the rope over a beam. She had called her case manager. She had also tried to hang herself in hospital when she had first been admitted in her teens. She was referred by her case manager because she had a long-standing delusion that she was the subject of a conspiracy. She had been on Clozapine for several years. However, unusually, she had a job as a shop assistant and was trying to complete a diploma in information technology. At one point during the course of therapy, she went to university to study English. I ended up seeing her over the next 7 years or so. She used the opportunity of our first meeting to explain the things that troubled her.

Her long-standing delusion revolved around experiences of reference. This constituted the basic evidence on which her delusions seemed to be founded. She would interpret unexpected events as references to her. Often, she saw them as messages of some kind or as threats. She would interpret an event to be a reference to her, feel certain that this was right, and then fit it into her current conspiracy theory. The nature of the conspiracies had changed since she had first become psychotic at 17.

Currently she thought that she was being investigated by journalists who were going to make an expose about her, suggesting that she was a benefit fraud. She had seen other exposes in the press. Typically, this belief bothered her more when she was reminded of it by some coincidence. If she noticed something which seemed unusual, or out of place, she would interpret it in line with this conspiracy. In the past, she had had a series of delusions about political themes. She had believed that she had met people who were conspiring to take part in terrorist activities and that she had communicated with them as part of a conspiracy to carry out some terrorist action. She had gone on to believe that she was going to be a central figure in the conspiracy to start a bloody revolution which would be wholly negative in its

DOI:10.4324/9781003168379-14

effect. She had been admitted to hospital on several occasions after suicide attempts.

She was homosexual, although she had had a brief period in her teens when she used to date men. However, when I met her, she lived with her mother and had not had a partner since her teens. She was working, and had friends, most of whom she had made through hospital. She was also quite involved with a local human rights group and also knew some people through this. She talked quite easily and didn't find the process of engaging in therapy difficult. She didn't present her delusional ideas as problems, but it became clear that they significantly impeded her ability to progress in her life. The full impact of her delusions did not become clear for some time. As well as believing that there was a conspiracy against her, she would also become suspicious about people in a more general way, and this had had led to her losing jobs and losing friends. In fact, this was often more of a problem in that it led to her becoming increasing anxious, and this interfered with her ability to sustain a job. Her delusional ideas and suspicion had a major impact on her life. For example, she had not had a girlfriend for five years, mainly through this suspicion. At one point in therapy, she became convinced that the local human rights group were all talking about her behind her back, and although she had been going there for several years, she left.

She had her first psychotic breakdown while at school. At that time there were a few different stresses in her life that could have related to her breakdown. She had grown up in a middle-class home as an only child. Her mother had a job in the civil service and her father was a GP. She remembered some conflict between her parents and her father drinking. She said that there were often raised voices and often her parents slept in separate rooms. Her mother took responsibility for most of the things that needed doing. Theresa saw her mother as the head of the household. But most of the time she had felt safe. She had been encouraged to apply herself at school and she had had friends and had worked hard. She hadn't been top of the class, but she had been competent. Her parents were involved in the local community. When she was 12 her parents separated. She found this very traumatic. After this, she remembers feeling lost and her school work deteriorated. Her mother was a committed socialist and feminist, and political theme featured strongly in her psychotic beliefs.

She first became psychotic when she was 17 and had struggled after this, completing her studies from home with the help of her mother and returning to school to take her exams. Just prior to having the breakdown, she had had a relationship with a woman of her age that she had met through the human rights group. She felt the woman had been controlling and abusive. She hadn't had a relationship since then as she had found the experience quite confronting. (Later in therapy she also told me that she remembered a stranger exposing himself to her when she was a small child.)

She experienced thought broadcasting and thought insertion at this time. She believed that she had developed psychic powers and could influence events such as the weather, or car and plane accidents. She had been admitted to hospital a number of times sometimes after a suicide attempt and sometimes when she was floridly psychotic. Her main delusion at this time was that she had been discovered by a terrorist cell that was planning a bombing campaign. She had believed that she was being targeted by a maverick group who were planning a revolution. They wanted her to become a major figure in the upcoming revolution and the leader of the government once the revolution had occurred. She described the onset of the psychosis as very confusing and distressing. Over some time, she understood that she had been psychotic, but at first, she hadn't known what to make of it all. She had been consumed with feelings of guilt, which were reflected in her delusions.

She had regular meetings with a case manager at the beginning of therapy, although after a couple of years she was only seen by me and was occasionally reviewed by her GP. Her main medication was Clozapine. When she tried to cut this down, she became confused, anxious, and overwhelmed. One unfortunate side effect was that she gained weight. She worked casually as a shop assistant. She had been trying to complete an IT course so that she could apply for work with computers, but somehow found that she couldn't get it done. In the end, I saw her for many years. At the beginning, this was weekly but at the end it was once a month.

In the past, she has had a series of different delusions around political themes, but when she began psychological therapy she no longer had experiences of thought broadcast or insertion. And her delusion was more prosaic. She believed that there was a conspiracy to expose her as a benefit fraud. Although she didn't have a partner, she did have several female friends that she saw regularly. She hadn't had any counselling prior to being referred to us.

Therapy

Delusion Modification and Coping Skills Enhancement

In the first sessions, she presented her main goals as wanting to complete her degree and to find a partner. She had spent her 20s avoiding romantic relationships, for fear of being controlled and abused again but, now she wanted to settle down, she found that she wasn't able to meet anyone and time was running out. Following the principle of starting from where the client is, I didn't ask about her delusional ideas and they didn't come up in our discussion. However, it became clear that her delusions were a significant problem for her. It was very positive that she had not withdrawn into a delusional world, but over time it became clear that these beliefs had a decidedly negative and limiting effect on her functioning.

As well as believing that there was a conspiracy against her to expose her to shame and opprobrium by making an expose of her in the press. She also became suspicious of people in a more general way and this led to her losing jobs and leaving friends. For example, she became convinced that the leaders and some other members of the local human rights group that she had been a member of for several years were talking about her behind her back. And so she left and joined another group, and didn't see any of the people she had previously seen as friends. This sense of mistrust pervaded most of her relationships and activities. Often these suspicious ideas were not delusional, in that she was not sure that they were true, but this continuing level of suspicion most likely fed her delusional belief.

The first two months were focused primarily on building rapport, so I did a lot of listening, and I took a personal history. After this, we began to work cognitively on her delusion, because it emerged as a problem. I reframed her problems underlining the role of the belief in her other problems. I put it to her that her belief that there was a conspiracy to expose her in the papers caused her a lot of distress. She worried for days about being exposed in print. She worried that they would present her as a fraud and claim that she didn't have a right to her disability payments as there was nothing wrong with her. I suggested that if this belief was false, she was having this anxiety for no reason, so it would be worth checking this out. I pointed out that this made it hard to focus on work and other positive things in her life. This is the standard cognitive therapy line on setting up a contract to investigate the truth or falsity of a delusion. It's a helpful way to come at this as it doesn't insist that the client is wrong but it puts that possibility on the table, amongst other possibilities. This is likely to be seen as a respectful way of bringing this up. It doesn't demean the person or directly invalidate them as an agent. In suggesting that the client is capable of coming to their own conclusions about things, it sets up a collaboration. She agreed to examine the truth of the delusion. As she already accepted that she had a "psychiatric illness" I set up the alternative hypothesis that she got to think this way due to this "psychiatric illness"/ emotional problems.

Her evidence for the conspiracy was numerous incongruous occurrences which she would believe related to her. For example, she saw some graffiti in the street that made some negative comment about the Government and she had the intuition that it had been put there for her to see. She was certain of this and only wondered what the intent of the message had been. Had they wanted to let her know that she is being watched? She rated her belief in the truth of this conspiracy at 100% on that particular day.

She agreed that it would be worth examining the delusion. Why would she agree to this? Was it because I persuaded her that it would be worth checking this out because if she was wrong, she had a lot of unnecessary suffering? But if I am certain that something is true, why would I check it out, even if I didn't want to believe it? More likely she agreed to check it out as I had suggested it to her, given that we had now something of a rapport, so that agreeing to check out the truth or falsity of the delusion follows from the development of a positive transference, rather than from a purely intellectual calculation.

We looked at whether the evidence was credible. In particular whether her delusional interpretations were consistent with other things that she knew to be true about the world. One example (discussed further later) was that she had received a letter addressed to "Tramps UK Ltd" as a message that she was a slacker and shouldn't be receiving benefits. She thought "Tramp" referred to her being work shy. She basically took her strong intuition that this was true as evidence that it was true. I set up the alternative hypothesis that this could be delivered in error. Some of the challenges to her paranoid interpretation of this event were: As the address on the envelope was not her address how would the person sending the letter know that it would get to her through the postal system? Why would whoever it was choose such a roundabout way of making these accusations? If they wanted to accuse her why not just come out and say so? Why not an anonymous letter making the accusations if they didn't want to be known? Other evidence included seeing graffiti which made some reference to crime in the street. She felt that this had been left for her as a message to her. I asked her how they would know that she was going to pass by at that time, as it wasn't a street that she frequently used? I introduced alternative explanations of these experiences or evidence as part of the "challenging" process. Although this sometimes had an effect on the degree of belief in the session, it did not lead initially to a sustained drop in her degree of belief. At times of stress, the belief would come back strongly, whereas if she was feeling calmer, it would generally be at the back of her mind. In the session, she would accept that the interpretation was probably not supported by the evidence, but the delusion did not really alter across sessions. As well as ideas of reference about being accused of being a fraud, she had also had experiences that seemed to relate to her old delusion of a political conspiracy. These had the theme of revolution, and her having a central role in this. So, for example, in one place that Theresa had lived, a woman (who lived above her) had birds that used to come and sit on her balcony. Theresa wondered if this was because the woman was a secret agent receiving messages by pigeon post.

I went on working with her challenging her delusion for the rest of the time that I saw her. One could think of some of this as "booster" sessions of cognitive therapy but, in reality, it was more like a years-long campaign to introduce an alternative perspective into her mind. Much of the time we dealt with other issues but when she became particularly bothered by a delusional idea, I would recur to challenging the evidence for this belief. Often this was when she was under stress of some kind. Although she didn't report that her delusional belief was abandoned, her degree of belief did drop. She said, years later, that that when she got a paranoid idea, she would imagine me questioning it, asking about the evidence and whether it was consistent with other things that she believed to be true. She found this approach to her delusion helpful. Another way of describing this is that at first the therapist acts like an external part of the client's ego, and over time this helpful external object is incorporated into the client's mind.

Trauma and Abuse

Recently the high incidence of trauma and abuse in psychotic client's childhoods has been emphasised and the importance of therapy for trauma and abuse in this group has also been highlighted (Read, 2018). In clinical practice, the appropriateness of this type of work needs to be assessed, including the client's ability to tolerate this kind of approach. The development of imagery rescripting methods (Smucker et al., 2021; Young et al., 2003; Young & Lindemann, 1992) has allowed trauma to be dealt with in imagery with much less danger of the client being re-traumatised. Sometimes, of course, memories of trauma can be delusional, but it is most helpful to assume that the memories are accurate unless there is clear evidence that this is not the case.

After about a year of therapy in which I had mainly focused on engagement, coping skills enhancement, encouragement, and challenging her delusion, the sessions moved into exploring her history of childhood trauma and abuse. Childhood trauma, in her case, was related to her difficulty in romantic relationships, with work, and with her ability to trust people in general.

Around the age of 7, a stranger in a park had sexually assaulted her. She had no idea what was happening but knew that it was wrong. She managed to find a way to let her mother know about this. Her parents responded in a supportive and protective way. She felt that they had taken effective action to keep her safe, and had allowed her to talk about her feelings without panicking or being overwhelmed, so she had got the feeling that she was supported rather than blamed and that it was a trauma that could be dealt with. Following this event, she began to act in a sexualised way towards other children. And she was left with guilty feelings about this.

One way of approaching these feelings would be to use a Gestalt therapy/Schema-Focused Therapy technique or imagery rescripting (Young et al., 2003; Young & Lindemann, 1992). Imagery receipting was developed as a method by Mervin Smucker (Smucker et al., 2021) as a way of working with traumatised clients who had been admitted to a psychiatric hospital. Paul Chadwick (2006) and John Rhodes (2022) give examples of using a modified schema therapy approach with psychotic clients. The client role plays a traumatic situation either in imagination or by imagining someone sitting in an empty chair. The therapist, in role play, can confront the abuser, coach the client to confront the abuser, and reimagine the trauma memory changing it so that the trauma is avoided or someone steps in to protect the client.

But I approached this by suggesting that we make the trauma the focus of our sessions, and left it to her to bring what she wanted to talk about.

This borrows something from the analytic technique of free association. Also, it is allowing her to set the pace and therefore avoids the possibility of the client feeling pushed into or compelled to do the imagery work. With clients who have been or are psychotic and who are therefore vulnerable, it seems important to approach these issues gently. The most important thing here seems to be to not make the client worse. By suggesting that we work on the trauma, I was offering an agenda or focus, but allowing her to take this up at her own pace. Obviously, I didn't know to what degree she could talk about the trauma without becoming overwhelmed. This is the issue of the so called "window of tolerance". Suggesting that we should use role play or imagery might have been overwhelming for Theresa, and this would be counter-therapeutic. She hadn't really talked about it before so suggesting that she might want to talk about it seemed a sensible place to start. She explained that when the abuse had happened, she had felt well protected by her parents. She said that some of her most upsetting memories were those of her acting out sexually with other girls, particularly one occasion when the other girl had become distressed. She worried what the parents must have thought of her. She felt that the experience of abuse had linked sexuality with hostility and she then feared her own response. Most of the work around the abuse consisted of listening to the narrative and re-interpreting the narrative in a non-judgemental and de-catastrophised, normalised way.

This early experience of sexual abuse had been reinforced at adolescence. As a 16-year-old she had had a girlfriend who was, very demanding. Looking back on this time she felt that she had been pushed around. It was around this time that she had her first breakdown. This made it difficult to be sure about what was real and what was illusion in some of the memories she had. If a client tells us a clearly impossible story about the past (e.g. that they had been present at the creation of the universe and had witnessed the big bang), it is easy to see that something is delusional. However, if someone tells us that someone was conspiring against them in a non-bizarre way, it is less clear. Theresa told me that her girlfriend had been conspiring to involve her in prostitution. Possibly this was delusional, or at least an overly suspicious account of what she was doing. Then again maybe this part of her account was true. Who can say for sure? Fortunately, we do not need to share our doubts with the client and developing rapport here is primary. Arguing with a client about what was or wasn't the case isn't going to get us anywhere. However, it was at this time that she began to think that she had caused bad things to happen by playing with an Ouija board. As mentioned earlier, she had stopped going to school and only completed her exams by being home schooled by her mother. She managed to get her GCSEs. She was admitted to hospital with grandiose delusions about being in touch with anarchist subversives. She gave up having relationships. Her experience had been that sex was linked with hostility and damage and that relationships were very similar. We talked about these events for several sessions and I wrote a letter to her summarising what had happened in a non-blaming way. She worried that she had caused damage to other children by acting out sexually. She felt that being sexually assaulted had made her more sexually aware. It seemed important not to minimise this and also not to demonise her for what she had done; that is to write the letter from a position of trying to understand her behaviour and her fears that the experience of being abused had turned her into a monster.

Final Stage of Therapy

After this, we moved onto the final stage of therapy which focused on whatever she would bring along as important current issues. This phase actually went on for several years. I didn't set an agenda. The client talked about whatever seemed relevant to her. Usually this was some personal problem, and I worked with her on understanding it. Often there would be an element of paranoia about her interpretations of events and I would be engaged in cognitive challenging (as described earlier). I linked themes of her current problems to those from her past and, also linked these themes to her relationship with me.

Conceptualisation

Theresa's initial breakdown in her teens occurred when she was struggling with issues around sexuality. She felt, she says, exploited by her girlfriend and she didn't trust her. Her early experiences of being abused set the stage for this, that is, for seeing sexuality as aggressive and dangerous. After this, she avoided relationships.

Her original delusion was that she would be involved in a clandestine terrorist/revolutionary movement. In this narrative, she is being manipulated into bringing about or being involved in things which are dangerous and likely to harm people. Also, she is to be in a major role in this situation. This is a type of concrete thinking or, if you like, unsignalled metaphor. She is uniquely bad and guilty. She is sought out by these terror groups, because she has special powers of being able to read minds and influence the future. She began to believe that her girlfriend wanted to lead her into prostitution. This is a regressed state of mind in which she is out of touch with reality and her world is populated by demons. The experience of splitting and projection affects the boundaries of her ego and the breakdown of the boundaries of the self leads to experiences of thought insertion and thought broadcast. She feels in danger from powerful forces outside of herself. This is also, of course, a grandiose belief. To be the woman who brings down the government and will be involved in bombings that will kill and maim is hardly self-esteem enhancing. This part of the delusion shows her taking a narcissistic stance. The world revolves around her, rather than her having a small part to play in the drama of humankind.

The delusion demonstrated the primitive psychotic defence of splitting and projection. Whatever the trauma that led to her breakdown once she has become psychotic, good and bad are clearly split. She has become identified with evil. She fears that good has been obliterated. The delusion that she had when I first saw her in her late 20s was less bizarre than this initial delusion. Then she believed that she would be exposed as a benefit fraud. The evidence for this was based on ideas of reference about seemingly everyday events. The cognitive conceptualisation here—that she was experiencing abnormal feelings of meaningfulness which she then interpreted as evidence for a conspiracy—seems viable, in as far as it goes. But it leaves unexplained where these delusions of reference come from. In this delusion, she will be seen as guilty and exposed to public stare. Both the earlier delusion and the later delusion centre on guilt. It isn't difficult to take this back to its historical origins in her childhood. Her solution to these feelings of fear and guilt was to avoid being in a relationship throughout her 20s. This solution, however, proves unstable as another part of her wants to love and be loved. She came into therapy in conflict. One part of her wanted to keep herself safe by withdrawing from relationships and life, and another, healthy, part of her wants to love and be loved.

This conflict becomes psychotic, however, when her thinking becomes concrete and she lacks of insight into these symbolic stories or images. This is an example of a changed mental state in psychosis, of a loss of boundaries. She has an idea which expresses her feelings about what has happened to her but confuses this idea with reality. Her experience of feeling that there is personal meaning in everyday events is a change in her "ego boundaries". She cannot differentiate between feeling guilty and being persecuted. The evil or bad is projected out into the people who want to harm her. At the same time, she will be exposed. In the more recent delusion (that she will be exposed as a fraud on TV) the content is more plausible. But the theme of the delusion is very similar. The delusion expresses the guilt but also neutralises it by externalising it. The persecution is from the outside, rather than internal. What has been internalised is a relationship between victim and persecutor so that this is also an expression of her as a victim, as when she was abused. This, then, is persecutory guilt rather than redemptive guilt.

A function of the delusion is defensive—to avoid the pain of the guilt. A cost is that she has split off and lost a part of her mind. The process of fitting the evidence to the belief takes place as documented in the cognitive account of delusions.

Cameron (1943, 1959) has described how this leads to an increasing withdrawal from other people so that a person ends up living in a world of their own. Clearly, Theresa was not in this situation. Psychosis involves withdrawal from the world of other people, but this process varies in degree between different people. If this psychodynamic account of her delusion is correct, the question raised whether working on testing the reality of the delusion using cognitive techniques is consistent with this. After all, if the delusion is a motivated defensive manoeuvre, or indicative of a regressed changed psychological state, then how could an approach based on the hypothesis that a delusion is essentially some type of mistake be helpful? Other people will have pointed out to the client that they're in error. This particular argument, however, is not confined to delusions or psychosis. A similar argument can obviously be made about, for example, phobias. Also, this argument can be made against psychodynamic interventions themselves. If an obsession, for example, is motivated by avoiding acknowledgement of an unacceptable impulse, why would interpreting this affect the obsession?

The main use of the psychodynamic conceptualisation is to try to understand where her relationships fit into this, and to understand the interaction between the therapist and client in terms of this. That, she regressed into a world peopled by good or bad characters. And she felt that she was possibly a bad character is important information. However, it must be remembered that she is no longer in that regressed state. She finds glimpses of it in her fears of being attacked and humiliated in the press, and throughout the sessions this is a repeated issue, but she also has functional relationships with her friends and family.

Transcripts

The following examples from transcripts of sessions illustrate the use of some of these ideas.

A Session

She arrived with a bag with the flag of the Soviet Union on it. I hadn't seen her and then I was 10 minutes late picking her up from the waiting room. I brought her a coffee and returned. I asked her if she had been in the waiting room for long. I offered to see her for extra 10 minutes. I asked her to rate her degree of conviction in the delusion (that she is being conspired against to publish an expose about her). She said that her conviction was currently low. Life was going well. She said that she was where she wanted to be. She is back at college. It was better than the first semester. She finds that she thinks about the paranoid thoughts but then asks herself "what would Simon say?" Its Simon says! I heard a woman say "I don't want anything to do with you" but I thought "I'm nowhere near her" (So that the comment couldn't have been meant for her). I bought a coffee and the man said "How is your day?" And I'm always wary of how to answer (because of being suspicious about what he will do with the information and why he wants to know) and I said "Ok". I heard him ask what a customer's name was and I thought "He can't even remember people's names . . . he doesn't know anything about me" (so that his inquiry was not sinister). Sitting on the bus, I was worrying about getting a reduced fare, because I'm on a pension. I get half price. And I thought "Hold on. I don't listen to the other people buying their tickets so why should they be listening to me". (So that the suspicious thought that other people would hear her ask for a reduced fare and inform on her for a benefit cheat was not true.) And I'm feeling better about the class. Because I've done a social welfare course, I could say that I know about Feminism or psychoanalysis. Not as in the same way as in literature but I still know, while other people say "I don't know anything". The English teacher was being positive about my essays. But I still have lunch on my own. She said that she had had some positive paranoid thoughts. She wondered if the teachers had changed the course to make it easier for her. I wonder if it's to do with being busy. "Idle minds are the Devil's playground. Do you know that expression?"

In this session, she has obviously internalised the therapist's questioning of her suspicious thoughts and describes the thoughts as paranoid. One explanation of this is that she has learnt a technique, but we could describe this as having internalised an aspect of her therapy. In any case, it is progress.

A Later Session

She arrived a little early. I arrived for the appointment and she was already there. Someone was in our room. I let her in and returned with two coffees. She said that she thinks about her paranoid beliefs every day, that they had only distressed her a little and that they were probably false. She had had a mixed week. She was happy studying at university. But she was really very distressed that she had lost her file of her handwritten creative essays somewhere on the campus. All her essays were in the file and she had written them out rather than typing them as she thought better that way, but she didn't have any copies. She had no idea where it was. She had been going to different places on the campus and ended up with 5 minutes to go before her bus left. She had gone to eat and not noticed that that she didn't have it. She didn't know why she hadn't realised. She had to get the bus to get to the evening job that she was doing. So, when she realised, she had to cancel the bus and go and look for the essay file. She couldn't find it. She thought that maybe some guys had found it. A lot of the stories were about intimate relationships so maybe some guys had found it and thought it was pornography and taken it. There was something odd going on with Subway. She had gone and asked had anyone left a folder of essays and the girl had said she'd get the manager. And he came out with a big smile and said to contact security. She had already done this. But she didn't like his smile. She thought that maybe he had stolen the file because of the stories being about sex. It wasn't the file itself as much as the essays. Then she broke into a big smile and said that on the other hand I'm really pleased with university. My teachers have been saying that my creative writing is good. One teacher said that I must have been writing before a lot (but actually I haven't). Did you read the essay I gave you last week?

I said that I had and said that it was very good.

She said that the ending of the story was a little ambiguous and at the end they had separated and not gone to bed together, had I understood that? What are you thinking? That's a serious look!

I said that maybe she was telling me about the ending so that I won't think that it's about sex. She said that that wasn't about sex but that her mother had read it and thought that they ended up in bed together, so she wanted to clarify this wasn't the case.

She then explained that she had gone to a socialist meeting and had been disappointed. At first, she had thought it was good but then a woman had asked her about what she was studying. She explained she was studying English and this had ended up in an argument about the nature of the texts and the portrayal of women in the texts. One of the texts that was on the curriculum was Lady Chatterley's Lover. The woman had said that she thought it portrayed women in a sexist way. One of the other members of the group said that he thought it was demeaning to women and that some of the books verged on pornography. Theresa had defended the book and asked what was wrong with pornography in any case? She thought to herself "How could they be so narrow minded?" I suggested that she had felt judged. She said "Yes. But this time I don't think that I was imagining it. Do you?"

Therapist:	If I suggested that everyone in the world was positive and not judgemental you would probably think that I was naive. They do sound a bit judgemental. But I think that there is an internal judge too, that condemns these ideas.
Client:	I thought "How could they be so narrow-minded". I mean isn't it supposed to be about being able to be who you want to be? Not being told that because you are a woman you have to live by rules made up by men?
Therapist:	And maybe you were wondering if I was judging you?
Client:	No.
Therapist:	Earlier when you wondered what I was thinking maybe you wondered if I thought the story was pornographic.
Client:	No. I wondered if you thought I was being boastful about my story. But I've known you a long time now and you must be the least judgemental person. What do I do about the socialist group? I was hoping to make friends.
Therapist:	If we meet people from a group who are judgemental or rude it's easy to assume that all the group are like that. So, if you meet someone who is a particular religion or colour who is lazy or something it's easy to assume that everyone from that group is. You could go back and talk to other people.
Client:	I was thinking of some other social group, maybe a book club, or I could try Amnesty or something for older people.
Therapist:	Nearer your age.

Client: Yes, I have had some "Simon Says" moments. I saw a chair with no one in it and I thought it had been put there for me.
Therapist: Who by?
Client: By the students as a message I should talk to that as I had no friends.

Commentary

In this session, Theresa rates her degree of belief in her delusion as low. However, in the account that she relates, she is full of suspicion. She feels surrounded by dishonest men who want to keep her file of stories for sexual motives. In this story, she feels exploited and misunderstood. None of these feelings are psychotic but they certainly have a paranoid, persecutory feel to them, and in this case, there are also the themes of being exploited sexually. I try to relate some of these feelings to me, and she denies that this is the case. She reports that she has been recalling our conversations to challenge the delusion. Underlying the delusion is the idea that the world consists of the good and the bad. The same reciprocal role that drives the delusion drives a lot of what she talks about in this session. There is someone around who will judge her.

A Later Session

Theresa rated her belief in her delusion as 70% and said that she thought about it twice a day.

She began by saying that she had got another package from Tramps UK Ltd. When it had arrived, she had put it straight in the post box. I asked her about the package and she explained that there had been a mistake in the address but that she still felt concerned about it. She said that she had been thinking that it could be a message about her not working, the way she felt the last time that she got one of these packages. I wondered if there might be alternative explanations. She said "Like what?" and I said that the parcel could have been delivered by mistake. If they had wanted to send her a message why did the parcel have the wrong address on it? And why didn't they just come out and make the accusation in a straightforward way, write her a note addressed to her accusing her of being a sponger? She listened to this and didn't agree or disagree with it. She then went on to talk about moving house and how she cannot move until later in the year. Then she asked me if I had heard of Stockholm syndrome? She had watched a TV programme about it. Did I know what it was? She said that it was named after a terrorist incident in which two of the hostages had gone on to marry terrorists. She said that it was linked to domestic violence. She went onto talk about being abused and how this had made her very aware of sex at a very young age. She had ended up feeling guilty about this. She said that talking about it makes a huge difference. It helps her not to feel guilty about it.

When she had been driving out of London, she heard the song "Born to run" twice on the Radio. It was the Springsteen song. Did I know it. It's a song about escape. She felt like it was about her getting away. She had felt like it was a message to her, about moving house and her going away. As she clearly meant this literally, we talked about what would be involved in sending her this message, how would they know she would be listening at that time? How many people would have to be involved? And in this case what would be the motive? She went on to talk about dealing with a lawyer about the conveyancing for the house she was buying. The lawyer didn't seem to be shocked that she was buying the house. She was in a class and there was a sign which said "Education is a right not a privilege". She felt that this message was there because she was in the class and the message was that she should get off her arse. I said that an alternative here is that because she feels guilty about not working, she sees things as messages about this as it's on her mind. I had previously given her the idea of confirmation bias. She had seen a woman in a wheelchair and a child with cancer. She felt really guilty about having disability payments herself. This, she felt, could be a message from the Universe. The meaning of the message is that she shouldn't fake being ill and needing long-term sick benefit when in truth there is nothing wrong with her.

At the beginning and the end of the session, she talks about her experience of meaningful coincidences and this comes up again at the end of the session. The background to this is that she is about to move house and feels anxious about this. One of her running anxieties is that people will think that because she isn't working, she has no right to a house. So, her anxieties about being attacked or rejected come up. In this context, the middle part of the session which looks, at first, as if it is unrelated to the rest of the session makes sense. It reminds her, probably unconsciously, of the feeling of guilt when she had been made aware of sex as a small child. I mainly listened to her talking, which she says is helpful and then engaged in some cognitive challenging. It would have been possible to make a link between her current feelings and those she had as a child.

A Much Later Session

Much later, she has stopped going to university and has started working. She had a job working as a book keeper. She had met a woman and started to date her. The next issue was going to be whether they should live together.

She arrived at the session looking flustered. She had messaged me to let her into the building, which was not supposed to be the routine. However, she usually did this so it wasn't unusual. She said that there were difficulties at work. One client who was very difficult she wasn't going to see anymore. She might apply for some other job. She was losing work due to reduced demand. It was all a bit up in the air. She had applied for a job but they hadn't got back to her, maybe because of the way things were going these days. She had just come from her mother's house. While she was visiting the police arrived and asked who lived there and took the details of who was there. There had been some reports of loud music and they were checking if there had been music being played at her mother's house. However, she went on to say that they thought that a neighbour had complained about them to the police because of a car parking dispute. She then went on with talking about her struggle with work with her relationship. Here there are indications of the progress that she has made. Obviously over 10-year therapy it is not possible to know what has produced change. Her preoccupations in this session are with her relationship to her partner and her difficulties at work. There are problems in both these areas but the incident with the policeman arriving at the house did not get interpreted in a delusional way. She did not think that the police were, for example, raiding the house because of a campaign about her, or to gather information about her. That she was preoccupied with her life difficulties rather than this incident does seem like progress. She has moved from preoccupation with her imagined persecutors to preoccupation with dealing with other people, and engagement with the world. When I made comments in the session she more or less ignored them and continued talking about her preoccupations. This is, obviously, less positive. She talks about being involved in her life, and not about the psychotic symptoms. However, in the session, the level of rapport is low and I am more or less ignored. At the end of the session, she said that she had been getting suspicious thoughts about her partner and about her family, which is again less positive.

A Later Session

This session was eight years into her therapy with me. By this time, she was attending once a month. She was in the process of getting a civil union with her partner, and prior to this she and her partner were buying a house together. She arrived at the office of her lawyer with her mother. Her partner had not transferred the money to the account as had been agreed. Theresa said that her mother and the lawyer were both anxious and were getting suspicious about what was going on. They were suggesting that her partner was behaving dishonestly. Theresa felt devastated. This was her worst fear. She left the meeting and drove onto a motorway and began driving. She didn't know where she was going. She eventually stopped the car and decided to go back. Although the idea was only half formed, she just wanted to escape from what she feared was the betrayal she had always feared and that others seemed to be confirming. What was in her mind was whether to not come back. She was able to conquer this impulse towards suicide. The other important thing here is that she didn't develop a paranoid interpretation of what had happened despite her mother and her lawyer giving her "evidence" that this was the case. She returned and it turned out that her partner had had cold feet and had some reservations and doubts but that she had eventually overcome these and had paid the money into the account, albeit it late. They had gone on to purchase the house and have the civil union as planned.

As her last relationship had been when she was 18, she found some aspects of her new relationship at 40 difficult. Then she had felt pestered for sex by her girlfriend more or less all the time. At 40, she found the fact that it was not like this now a little disappointing and she began to worry about whether her partner loved her or whether she might be asexual. However, the positive thing here was that she didn't retreat from the ups and downs of a relationship into a delusional world but tolerated the frustrations of their relationship. As well as the paranoid part of Theresa (that drove off down the motorway and that began to think that her partner might be asexual), there is also another part of her personality which enabled her to keep persisting with her relationship (and indeed with work or study). It is not just the experience of abuse that is important but the experience of care and love which allow the development of possible positive relationships with others or hope in the future.

The Beginning of Sessions

Often clients will begin a session with an interaction of particular relevance to the transference. This may be because at the beginning of the session the client is feeling disturbed by the process of reconnecting to the therapist, because breaks in treatment are unconsciously associated with other breaks and disturbances in other relationships. In any case, events which trigger possible paranoid, or negative, perceptions of the therapist are particularly useful in therapy, as illustrated by the following example.

As Theresa walked towards my office, we passed a nurse from the pathology clinic who said "Hello". After we sat down, Theresa looked perplexed. I asked her what was going through her mind and she said that it seemed strange that the nurse had said "Hello". I explained that I knew the nurse as she worked next door in the pathology clinic, which was why she had smiled. Theresa had felt that it had meant something about her. She relaxed when I gave her this explanation. I asked her if she thought that this happened outside of the setting with me in day-to-day events, where she couldn't ask to find out why something unexpected had happened. Here I dealt with this paranoid interpretation in a matter-of-fact way by revealing something about myself. This had the effect of not just explaining the experience in a non-threatening way but also linking the experience to other possible experiences outside of the therapy. If I hadn't done this, her suspicions would probably have grown. The vicious cycle of paranoia involves the person interpreting things in a paranoid way, and then distancing him or herself from others because of fear but then reducing exposure to alternative explanations and therefore strengthening the account. It seems likely that it is the trusting relationship with the therapist that is central in allowing alternative explanations to be considered, and this is based on positive transference.

A similar situation occurred with the same client much earlier in the therapy. She had been in the waiting room in the psychotherapy department. While waiting, she had seen a nurse who was usually based in the Clozapine clinic but who was visiting someone in the department. At the beginning of this session, she had said that she had recognised the nurse and wondered what she was doing here. She went on to say that when she had been at the Clozapine clinic, she had felt that the nurse knew things about her that she had talked about with me in our sessions. In our most recent sessions, we had been talking about her history of child sexual abuse. I asked her if she wondered if I had talked to the nurse about what she had said to me. She answered in a way that left open the possibility either way. I explained that I didn't talk about what she said during the sessions to other workers. I reflected that it seemed difficult to trust me at the moment. She said that of course she trusted me.

The situation is the same in a number of ways. There is another woman who she suspects knows something about her and who has a relationship with me that threatens the confidentiality of our relationship. The implication is also that I have betrayed her trust, although she denies this. I drew attention to her lack of trust and the interpretation of the other woman as having knowledge about her so that I had betrayed her confidence. This is particularly useful in therapy because the central problem is occurring in the here-and-now of the relationship with the therapist. One of the factors which perpetuates a delusion is withdrawal from others which removes alternative explanations. So being able to address this interpretation in the presence of the person one is paranoid about sets the stage for building up an alternative hypothesis. Both of these examples occurred immediately before a session, when the client was in the process of reconnecting to me. She had similar experiences in many different places so an advantage here is that I could examine her suspicious interpretations in the moment and hope to clarify that the interpretation is incorrect while it is still new. In Theresa's case, this manoeuvre was successful. As I mentioned earlier, with a different client, my explanation would just be seen as part of the plot. If this is correct that the chance of altering a paranoid interpretation in a therapy session is higher the stronger the emotional bond between the therapist and client.

The Challenge of Living Together

I had not seen Theresa for several months. Once she had begun seeing her partner, she felt less need to attend the sessions. In some ways, she felt that the problem she came with had been resolved. I suggested that it was a good idea to keep coming to therapy as committed relationships, I suggested, as well as being a positive achievement, were also a period of upheaval and change. Probably the sessions had provided the opportunity to talk through her feelings and this felt less necessary once she had a partner. She and her partner had decided that before they moved in together, they would get a Civil Union (which had only recently been established for gay couples in the UK.) However, as the prospect of moving in together got closer some of her old anxieties recurred.

She had gone to the pharmacy to collect her medication and the pharmacy staff had been talking and laughing loudly together. She felt that they were laughing about her. This experience of feeling that others were talking about her is a recurring one. I came to believe that this was the central experience that drove her other paranoid beliefs. She became increasingly annoyed and agitated. She had given her prescription in but left without collecting it. The following day she had returned to pick it up. She had told the pharmacist that she hadn't been happy that the staff had been talking and laughing and the owner of the shop had apologised that she hadn't felt that they had dealt with her in the proper way. She had felt that they were talking and laughing about her because they had been dispensing a psychiatric medication to her, so she felt exposed and ridiculed. There would be a number of possible ways of taking this up with her, which are well described by Malan's triangles. There is her increased anxiety due to becoming closer and more committed to her partner, so her anxieties here can be addressed as reflecting her fears about being closer to her partner and the risk that this involves. Or, it could be taken up with reference to her relationship with the therapist. As she has been seeing me far less often this would possibly focus on her feelings of disconnection in relation to me. It could also be addressed in relation to her past. Her fears of getting closer to a woman dated from her teenage experiences with her girlfriend and to her earlier experiences of being sexually abused. However, the technical difficulty here is that she doesn't recognise that her reaction is paranoid. Her feeling of being abused or exploited is experienced as the perception that people in the pharmacy are laughing at her. Here it is important for the therapist to be aware that this perception relates to her fears about her current relationship and that this symptom (her paranoid reaction to the workers in the chemist) is a repetition of a past trauma, and that this relates to the reduced contact with the therapist and to the increased commitment to her fiancée. In many ways, she had established an equilibrium in living alone, and the prospect of living together was disturbing this.

I took up her fears about the particular incident at the pharmacy. Until she was clear that they had not been persecuting her as there was little point in relating it to me, or to her partner or to the distant past. I reflected that she felt that they were mocking her and I wondered what alternative explanations there might be. I suggested that one possibility was that she was right about the staff laughing about her and mocking her. But that there were other possibilities. We went through what these might be. She might be correct; she might be feeling anxious as things were changing in her life. This explanation was deliberately vague about what it could be that would be making her anxious. She agreed that she had been feeling anxious recently. This is a cognitive strategy, and helped her to step back from the experience and see her explanation as one amongst a number of explanations rather than as the only explanation. This particular intervention—taking a recent experience of reference and generating alternative explanations—can be helpful in loosening the person's attachment to just one explanation.

Earlier in the therapy, I observed how these delusions of reference could be very destructive to her life. On two or three occasions, she got a job and would get the idea that someone at work didn't like her and this would end up with her leaving the job. In the past, Theresa had taken a creative writing class at a local university. She wrote a story that was related to sexual abuse and then felt uncomfortable when other students commented on this aspect of the story. She began to feel that the other students were talking about her behind her back. She had been in a particular human rights group for many years and had socialised with the other members of the group. Eventually she began to think that the senior members of the group were talking about her. One of the members of the group was also a psychiatric nurse in the hospital she had been admitted to, which she found a little uncomfortable. Eventually she decided to leave. It wasn't clear what had led to this but she went to a different group in a different town and cut all contact with them. Later when she saw members of the group, she would think that they were where she was to spy on her. This pattern of suspicion leading to feeling that there was a conspiracy against her recurred and its effect was to isolate her. She moved to a new neighbourhood. Her next-door neighbour left some of his pornographic magazines outside his door in a bag. She felt sure that this was a signal to her. Her therapy functioned as a place to detoxify these paranoid ideas as they occur. Ideally in relation to the therapist (that is in the transference). I think that with Theresa, this was less that she had a belief which we tested to see if it was true, but more like building up the side of her that could doubt the belief.

A Later Session

Theresa had not come for a month. She looked quite serious. She said that she had two things on her mind that she would like to talk through. One was to do with her job and the other to do with her relationship. She said that she wasn't happy about her job. She said that the work is casual so there is no sick pay or holiday pay. She was going to look for another job. She has been there for two years and is paid at the casual rate. She said that she was just letting me know about the change. She then went on to talk about her relationship. She asked me if I had seen *Suspicion* by Hitchcock. I said that I had. She continued talking, not looking at me directly but slightly off to my right. She had recently seen it and it got her thinking. The woman falls in love but it turns out that her husband has been dishonest about his finances and his job and about his feelings. I suggested that she found this disturbing and that maybe she was worried about her own relationship. She didn't answer this comment directly but said that they had had some sexual difficulties, and this had happened since they had moved in together.

I said that maybe she was worried that her partner didn't love her. She said that the sex was different to the way it had been with her previous relationship. Then she and her girlfriend had been sleeping together all the time.

I said something about how she had been much younger, but she ignored this and went on to say that, if the relationship failed, it would be a disaster. She had taken out loans to buy the house. I suggested that she worried that her girlfriend didn't love her, and had only moved in with her as a convenience, like in the movie. She told me that she had ordered some books on sex from a local bookshop. Two of the books had arrived but the other book hadn't come. They had been waiting a couple of weeks. She was passing the shop and went in to buy a cookbook as a present for a friend. While she was paying for the present, she asked the shop assistant about the book which hadn't arrived. The shop assistant hadn't said anything. When she got home, there was a message to say that the book was coming. She said, with some feeling, that this seemed like quite a coincidence. I asked her what she thought was going on? She said that she thought that the book might have been delivered because she had visited the shop. Maybe, she wondered, they sent her the book because she had brought a cookbook and it was a message that she couldn't have the sex book until she had learnt to cook. I wondered about why, in that case, she had been sent the other two books about sex? She ignored this and went on to say that she also wondered whether some of her other experiences had damaged her: for example, looking at pornography. I pointed out that she would need a new referral before the next session and she said that she would get one from the GP. She found that the GP had a weird attitude. I asked in what why. She said that the GP had queried the need for a new referral and wondered what I was on about. Another strange thing had been that when she had been using her phone some adverts had come on about a particular type of car. It had been the type of car that she had been in one time when she attempted to kill herself (she had tried to kill herself by driving off the road). This, she thought was a message to remind her that they knew about her past mental illness and how bad she had been. Some of the older people in the human rights group had also been making comments, innuendos, about her and girlfriend. One man had said that now they were official that they should think about having children. They were not getting any younger. She had felt they were being monitored.

As the session ended, I suggested that we needed to be seeing each other more frequently as she had been feeling more paranoid, and she agreed with this.

In this session, maybe ten years after we began therapy, she is plagued by fears about her changed situation. All the anxieties that have kept her out of relationships have re-emerged. She wonders if her partner has moved in with her to get her hands on her money and is unable to really love her. She worries that she is being monitored and sent critical messages in a coded way to influence her behaviour. At the beginning, she more or less asks for reassurance that it is ok to talk about her relationship with her partner with me (I thought that she felt it slightly disloyal). She is surrounded on all sides by threats and critical messages. Her inner critic is externalised and guilt and fear come to her not as ideas or feelings but as external concrete sources of danger. She finds it hard to trust not just the GP but also her partner, and she feels as if every coincidence is proof of a sinister conspiracy against her. She is penned in. When I offer alternative perspectives, her main strategy is to ignore what I say and carry on talking, so she effectively turns a blind eye to disconfirming evidence, because she knows that it isn't true before she examines the evidence. She no longer trusts the GP. And this pattern has happened with most people that she has had contact with. She moved on from her previous political group and has given up several friends because of suspicions. I asked her if she ever wondered about me and she said that she didn't. The conditions of psychotherapy (confidentiality and non-intervention) allowed Theresa to have less doubts about me. This allowed her to talk freely about her concerns (as she said at the beginning of the session). This, of course, is quite an important role for a person whose emotional disorder leads them to being increasingly cut off from others. The fears that she expresses here are familiar from the early sessions that I had with her. In one way, nothing has changed. This is to say that cognitive therapy and maybe other therapy doesn't cure psychosis but can work to ameliorate it. In one way, she is an example of a failure to alter the tendency to interpret events with heightened feelings of reference. In a more important way of course, she is a great success as she is working, socialising, and having relationships.

In psychodynamic terms, Theresa has a persecuting inner parent. Much of the time this "inner object" is projected out and experienced as an external persecuting "object". This is based on her experiences of being abused (first by a stranger and then her experiences with her first girlfriend). However, acting out sexually with other girls also adds to this pattern and gives her a reason for fearing that she will be attacked. She is not bothered by feelings of guilt because these feelings are projected out into the environment and experienced as persecution.

Another notable feature of Theresa's experiences is the tendency towards concretisation. She experiences things in her environment as full of meaning directed towards her. She confuses feeling that something is the case with its being the case. Her fear that others will judge her is experienced by her as other's judging her. And the externalisation of guilt also involves a degree of concretisation, feeling she is faced with an enemy. She loses the boundary between herself and others, or the material world. Coincidences in the world are seen as significant because she feels herself to be at the centre of events, everything is arranged for her.

Furthermore, she elaborates the feeling of fear by imagining the worst possible outcomes, which makes her more fearful and this in turn makes her more sensitive. She experiences the advert for the car as meaningful because events in the world and events in her mind are not differentiated. The message is a warning from someone, although it isn't quite clear who. In this session, she expresses distrust in most of the people in her life, although she doesn't mention me. I felt mainly like I was excluded from the room and reduced to the role of listener, probably as a way of rendering me safe.

This regression into a more paranoid state of mind is related to a perceived threat, entering into a more committed relationship. It would be possible to address the increase in delusional ideas through an information processing model. However, it would also be possible to relate how she is feeling to the circumstances precipitating these experiences and to strengthen that link would be to enhance insight. The position of the therapist in the transference is important. She distrusts everyone. This is not aimed at me, but I feel she distances her contact with me (by avoiding eye-contact and by excluding the possibility of dialogue. This makes it unlikely that any intervention will be heard and that it is better to wait.

A Later Session

In a later session, Theresa continued with the same issue. She explained that it was difficult to talk about some of the things that had been going on. She explained (I think partly to herself) that she couldn't talk to anyone else about some of these issues. She looked at the ground and clearly found it very difficult to talk. She would begin to discuss a topic and then break off in the middle of what she was saying. She began by talking around the issue. She didn't want to make her partner feel bad about things. Maybe she had made a mistake in committing to someone. If it didn't work out then it would be difficult. She didn't want to be demanding. I commented that she had some concerns about the physical side of her relationship with her partner and she was disappointed about this and worried about it. She ignored this comment and carried on talking about her worries and not wanting to upset her partner. I felt that my comments were something of an intrusion. Eventually she got on to saying that they had gone on holiday together and that she had taken the book on sex. She had suggested that she should read it to her. They had had sex but she found it underwhelming. She began to read to her but quite quickly her partner said that she was feeling tired and went to sleep. Theresa had lain in the dark for a while and began to cry. I said that she felt disappointed and didn't know what to do. I said that sex in middle age isn't the same as it is when one is a teenager. She felt that she didn't know what to do and that talking about it seemed too difficult. She said that she felt really bad feeling like this and having these thoughts. I said that she felt unhappy but wasn't allowed to say so for fear of hurting her partner.

She then went on to tell me that she had heard them talking on the TV about her and her partner's problem. I asked her to describe what had happened. She said that the commentators on the TV had been making references to sexual difficulties in an indirect way and this had made her feel more uncomfortable. I asked her how that could work. I said as she hasn't told anyone about this how could they know about it? She said that maybe her partner had mentioned it to someone. She hadn't asked him about this though. I went on to talk with her about the alternative competing hypotheses of the TV presenters knowing about her and dropping hints versus her seeing the hints when they weren't there because she is sensitive to that issue at the moment. Here one of her anxieties gets reflected in the discourse of other people. She hears the issue she is feeling anxious and devastated about reflected in the conversation of others. Her preoccupations colour the messages that she hears implied in what she takes as hints. Her anxious preoccupations return to her from the outside in the mouths of the TV presenters. The experience expresses her feelings. Her feelings have been subjected to a type of concretisation by being turned into a perception. And she is not able to conceal what has happened in her private life. Clearly the psychotic experience has in some sense been produced by the conflict that she is experiencing. In other cases, it can be suggested that the psychotic experience has caused the fear or anxiety but in this case the feeling is separate from the psychotic experience and is expressed in the experience. The psychotic experience is an expression of the feeling as a perception.

A Later Session

For much of this session, it was difficult to engage in a dialogue with Theresa and rapport was low. She would begin talking and then go off at various tangents. She said that she was doing well. She will be going into the office more. It's the first time that she has worked full time since her new job as an IT worker. She has been doing a variety of things. She had been responding to calls for advice and help. She had also been involved in talking to some of the workers about how to get the best from the software that was newly available. She had applied for a job as a manager which was really very ambitious and unlikely that she would get it and they had offered her this other job.

There were some difficulties in the office. A client had been a bit inappropriate on the phone. She had been making small talk with the client on the phone and he had said something about his trousers. She had told her boss about this and the client had wanted to apologise to her. Later she had heard one worker laughing with another and saying "It must have been really scary staying in the kitchen" She had taken this as a reference to her (for reasons that I had trouble following). I suggested that she had a tendency to become overly suspicious and this could be one of these occasions; however, this was mistimed as she just insisted that she knew that she was right about this, despite not being able to identify any evidence.

References

Cameron, N. (1943). The paranoid pseudo-community. *American Journal of Sociology*, *49*(1), 32–38.

Cameron, N. (1959). The paranoid pseudo-community revisited. *American Journal of Sociology*, *65*(1), 52–58.

Chadwick, P. D. (2006). *Person-based cognitive therapy for distressing psychosis*. West Sussex and Malden, MA: John Wiley and Sons.

Read, J. (2018). Making sense of and responding sensibly to psychosis. *Journal of Humanistic Psychology*. *59*, 5.

Rhodes, J. (2022). *Psychosis and the traumatised self*. London: Routledge.

Smucker, M., Reschike, K., & Kogel, B. (2021). *Imagery rescripting and reprocessing therapy*. Berlin: Shaker.

Young, J. E., Klosko, J. S., & Weishaar, M. E. (2003). *Schema therapy: A practitioners guide*. New York: Guilford Press.

Young, J. E., & Lindemann, M. D. (1992). An integrative schema-focused model of personality disorders. *Journal of Cognitive Psychotherapy: An International Quarterly*, *6*(1), 11–23.

13 Tina

A Mid-Life Crisis

Tina was referred to the Bankstown Psychology Team by her psychiatrist. She was in her 50s and lived with her 25-year-old daughter. She had married in her early 20s and had been divorced for 12 years at the time that I met her. Tina was referred following an attempt to hang herself. Following the suicide attempt she had been admitted to the psychiatric ward and had stayed there for some months. When she was discharged, she was referred to the community team.

She had been working as a salesperson but had taken sick leave following a fight at work. She had been suffering from depression for some time. She had subsequently been dismissed. Her daughter was also not working, and she had got into arrears with her rent payments. This had increased her depression and anxiety and she had begun to feel that everything was hopeless. She didn't have a current partner. She presented with the following problems. She had been depressed for 18 months. This had led to her difficulties paying her rent. Her mood was low. She felt sad quite a lot of the time, had trouble sleeping and concentrating. However, she wasn't at all slowed down and she looked after her appearance and was able to engage in a dialogue in therapy. She cooked for, and generally looked after her daughter. She didn't really know why she had become depressed but she said that it was exacerbated by her unemployment, and inability to pay the rent. She worried about losing the house and being evicted. She had long-standing low self-esteem. She felt that she had been very good at her work, but outside of work she had low self-esteem. She had not had a partner for many years. She had dated a few men but these relationships had led to her being rejected. Her ex-husband had recently moved back into the house on a temporary basis as he had lost his job. He had a new partner, and was clearly not interested in her.

Tina said that she drank too much. Her daughter also drank to excess and would invite her friends around to the house and, when she had an audience, she was sarcastic to Tina. She found this set of unhappy events depressing and she felt she had little hope for the future. She had no job or partner and her home was under threat. Her daughter was publicly contemptuous of her.

DOI:10.4324/9781003168379-15

She had a long-standing delusion, with experiences of reference but no other psychotic symptoms. She thought her delusion was a positive discovery for her rather than a problem. She believed that people communicated in a secret language which she had hitherto not understood. People spoke with secret meanings. As well as the surface meaning of a statement there was sometimes a symbolic meaning, which was often related to sexuality. She also thought that she had begun to be able to communicate with people telepathically, and that many other people could also do this. Generally, she did not find the experience of hearing people talking with secret meanings distressing and no one was trying to harm her. Rather she felt that she was an outsider whose lack of understanding had contributed to her husband leaving her, her failures with men and the general contempt that others had for her. She took comments that others had made in the past to the effect that she lacked skills in talking to men and that she should learn how to communicate better as evidence that this was true.

She had been born in the 1960s to a working-class family. Her father had been a merchant sailor and she remembered her father always going away to sea. Her parents got on well and she was the youngest of three children. She said that it was an old-fashioned household at the time and that she grew up in an Edwardian atmosphere. Her parents were caring and treated her well, although as a child she didn't feel emotionally close to either of them. She couldn't talk about her problems with them. She had enjoyed some things about school, but she had had dyslexia and had struggled to learn to read. This had had a negative effect on her self-esteem. She remembered having to read out passages in class and failing, and being placed in special classes for people with a learning disability. She was bullied about this by the other schoolchildren. Her feelings of low self-esteem seemed to originate in these experiences. She had a large extended family who lived nearby and there were often parties. She remembered members of her family making fun of her difficulty in reading. She felt that she was unacceptable wherever she went. Her parents tried to help her by encouraging her to not take the mockery to heart. She remembered trying not to read or write to avoid being made fun of. In the year before she left school, she became more outgoing and sociable but before this she had been unhappy throughout her childhood. She had left school at 15 years and got whatever work she could find. She had two relationships with men. She fell pregnant with her second boyfriend and gave birth to their daughter and they married two years later.

When her daughter was three Tina found work as a salesperson. In this job, her difficulty with reading and writing wasn't a problem and she was good at dealing with the customers. When she was in the role of a salesperson she found that she could be full of confidence, unlike in her personal life. She was quite successful at selling. This had been the happiest time of her life; when she was in her early 30s, she lost both her parents within a year of each other, and she became more distant from her sister and brother. She had seen them increasingly less after her daughter was born.

An important event in her life occurred a few years later when she was in her mid-30s. She and her husband had gone on holiday with another couple. She began to feel that her husband was having an affair with the other woman. She had accused him of this and he had denied it, but she continued to believe that he had been unfaithful to her. She had begun to believe that he was communicating in a secret code with the other woman. She heard double meanings in what he said. This was the beginning of her delusional belief, and she had first seen a psychiatrist at this time. A couple of years later they separated and divorced. He maintained that she had been crazy. When they divorced, her ex-husband got remarried but not to the person with whom she had suspected him of being involved with.

Her daughter, who was 12, however stayed with her so she brought her up as a single parent. She had two further relationships which did not work out. Around this time, she lost her older brother. She had looked to him for advice, rather than her father, so this was a painful loss. However, it was some 8 or 9 years after that she became depressed in her early 50s. Her depression occurred in the context of mid-life issues. She began to feel that she was going to be on her own, and not find a permanent partner and her daughter was now an adult and making her own way in the world, albeit in Tina's house. These troubles probably precipitated her depression. Around this time, she had become more preoccupied with the idea of hidden meanings in what people said. It is clear that she was faced with a personal crisis. Her daughter had grown up and didn't need her mother's care and they had a difficult relationship. She had not made a successful new relationship so her role in her family had disappeared and she hadn't replaced it with another. She was facing growing older on her own. She had still worked until recently but she took no pleasure in life. And then she lost her job.

The delusional belief that other people spoke with a secret language that she had never understood, and that she could communicate telepathically strengthened. These delusions were largely based on changed experience of the world. She thought that everyone else understood this way of speaking and only she had been unaware of it. Discovering this had been something of a revelation to her. The secret communication consisted largely in hidden, symbolic meanings and allusions. She thought that this explained the breakdown of her marriage. Her husband had been communicating with hidden meanings to his lover while she was with them. In fact, it explained all of the failures in her life. Her husband and his lover had used double meanings and codes, to set up meetings together. The insight that she had into her life was that she had been lacking in a basic skill in communication in relationships. This explained why she was alone. She had a defect. She couldn't understand how men and women talked to each other. Now she could hear the double meanings and also now she could communicate telepathically. This belief symbolised the cause of her problems. She was defective and unable to talk to men in a way that would be attractive, so it barred her from relationships. It wasn't her that was the problem it was the lack of a particular skill. It also implied that other people had used her defect against her. No one had told her about it plainly and her husband used her lack of understanding to have an affair under her nose. Unfortunately, it also led to her misinterpreting a comment from a co-worker and that led to her getting into a fight at work. This meant that at the age of 55 she lost her job and had then attempted to hang herself, and was admitted to hospital. The financial crisis that losing her job produced- she could no longer afford the mortgage—had deepened her depression and precipitated the suicide attempt.

Therapy

This began with an initial four weeks of listening and engagement, followed by a period of behavioural/solution-focused work on her low mood and finally with an attempt to modify her delusional belief.

Engagement

I began therapy with her with engagement- a period of listening and taking a personal history over a period of about a month. During this time, I had her rate her degree of belief in the delusion. She was absolutely convinced that her delusional belief was true.

Cognitive-Behavioural Stage

As her main problem from her point of view was low mood, I asked her to record situations in which her depression was worse. She returned with a series of situations. The thoughts or meanings associated with being more depressed included (1) not having a partner, (2) hearing people say things that had a double meaning, (3) being out of work, and (4) being put down by her daughter. The underlying meaning, revealed by the downward arrow technique, was of being a failure. Her delusion is an unacknowledged symbolic expression of this failure. So, if one function of the belief was to protect her self-esteem it ultimately was unsuccessful. Here her sadness about her life, about being alone and not being in work add to her sense of personal inadequacy. She felt, however, that although she now understood the special communication people used it was too late for her to change. In particular, this seemed to relate to the series of broken relationships she had had. It also became clear through her diary keeping that her problem with her daughter was quite difficult. (Mid-way through the therapy her ex-husband and the mother of her daughter had moved back into the house as she had had nowhere else to go. But this was a purely practical arrangement and she had no interest in Tina.) She found the combination of her daughter putting her down and having her ex-husband in the house doubly difficult. Both of these things added to her feeling of low self-esteem.

Actually, it became clear later that she also had fears for her sanity. She had absolute conviction that she was correct in there being double meanings in things that people said. She also believed that she could communicate telepathically with people. But after I had been seeing her for a while, she let me know that she feared that she might be losing her mind, which implies that another part of her was aware that she might be in error. Here is one of the motives for certainty about a delusion. "If I am wrong about this then maybe that means I am crazy". The symptom (the delusion) is maintained by the defensive mechanism of denial to defend against the anxiety of being mad.

We worked on her relationship with her daughter. For many years it had been just the two of them. Now her daughter drank every night and sometimes invited her friends around. When her friends were there, she would make jokes at her expense. Tina found this made her feel very uncomfortable, and it reminded her of being mocked by her extended family as a child, and bullied at school. If her daughter was sober, or if she didn't have an audience, there were no problems. I asked her what she had tried to deal with this problem. She had suggested that her daughter should move in with her father or that she should get a job and move out into a flat of her own. Her daughter was 25 and had not worked since she left school. She had no friends of her own age but had friends who were still at school. One solution, she said, would be to keep the kids out of her house. She had tried to put her foot down but her daughter didn't listen to her. I took this up in therapy and we used role play to practice an assertive response to her daughter. She wasn't sure that this would help. At the next session, she said that she had felt low most of the time and that she had tried to talk to her daughter but that it hadn't worked. She talked about how her difficulties in reading and writing made her feel negative about herself. She said, with some emotion, that she couldn't have a proper relationship as she had sexual difficulties. She had not followed up on the suggestion that she should try to an alternative way of responding to her daughter but, on the other hand, she had talked more about her personal problems in the session so this indicated a deepening sense of rapport, so that this was a success. She also talked about her own aggression. Her ex-husband, who had returned to the family home made things more difficult for her by taking her daughter's side. She felt pushed out and challenged by her daughter who acted like it was her house. Although we were no nearer to any solution to her problems it was clearer that she felt inadequate as a woman and that other people were hostile and mocking. This theme, of course, was present in the history she gave of being mocked at school and by her family about her dyslexia. Her delusion in fact seems a symbolic expression of her particular difficulties with communication and relationships with people. Tina had no insight into this link.

She said that her divorce had been her husband's idea and that he had told her that she "needed help". It is possible that her jealous accusations against her husband led to the breakdown in the marriage. If so then it would have been another example of a paranoid belief leading to social withdrawal and alienation, partly by its effect on other people. The hostile and rejecting part of her is projected into her husband who acts it out towards her. Fearing the loss of her husband's love she reacted in a hostile way which had contributed to alienating her husband until he tells her he wants a divorce and that she "needs help", confirming that she is unlovable and that others are rejecting and cruel. She said that she thought that her problem in these situations was that she took things to heart.

She complained of losing her temper. Working from a solution-focused position, I asked her for exceptions to this. She said that watching comedy shows on TV helped. Continuing with this line of therapy, I asked her to notice (1) when things went well and (2) when she managed to avoid a fight at home. At the next session, she said that she felt at a standstill. The mortgage needs to be paid and she had no job. She was worried that she would have her house repossessed by the bank. She had not been having unpleasant interactions with her daughter. She had tried to talk to her about the problem. Although most of her identified problems were still present her mood improved.

I asked her the "Miracle Question". If there were to be a miracle and her problem was resolved overnight, how would she know on waking the next day? She said that she would notice that she would feel a bit lighter and would be smiling and joking with people. I suggested that she might try and act like this. At the next session, she told me that she had been putting it into practice. She had got up earlier in the morning and tidied up the garden. Also, her daughter had been drinking less. She said that she used to feel small with people. Now she was able to ignore it. Her daughter's friends had come around but were not being so outlandish. She noticed that her mood was better now that the place was tidy.

At the beginning, the therapy was the same as it would be if she had not had a delusion. As cognitive therapy is collaborative, it is much more straightforward to get to collaborate on problems that both the client and the therapist agree exist. As the sessions progressed, I began to talk more with her about her experiences of the secret language, double meanings and telepathy. She told me that she was feeling less depressed. She had previously been worrying that the neighbours were watching her. She had been feeling self-conscious and had been worried if anyone had spoken to her. She had been worrying that she was losing her mind. This phenomenon is important. As she has begun to trust me more, she is able to tell me more of her experiences and feelings. In a brief cognitive therapy, such as this, we are half way through treatment before certain important aspects of the problems are available for discussion. But this is not necessarily a case of a client having a secret which they keep from the therapist. (Although, obviously, that can and does happen.) When Tina began to talk to me about her suspicions about the neighbours and her fear that she was going insane, sharing this with a therapist demonstrated an increasing trust in me and being clearer in her own mind about some of her fears about her mind, so rapport is heightened, and, given that her core problem is in trusting others, this progress in the transference is a significant gain. Nothing has been interpreted here, but it is important that the therapist is aware of this as, otherwise, it might seem that the client is little improved. This raises a technical difficulty, one that occurs frequently with in working with psychotic clients. She feels relieved that she is not going insane, but as her therapist I didn't feel so sure and also, of course, whereas she felt that her experiences of telepathy were insights I thought that they were psychotic experiences.

How to handle this involves a risk assessment. It's helpful if the client has a case manager who can take the lead on managing these concerns which reduces the pressure to address this in therapy. Tina didn't have a case manager. How stable the symptoms are is an important factor. In Tina's case, the beliefs and experiences had been present for some time. Although she didn't have a case manager, she did have psychiatrist who saw her regularly. If one is the only person reviewing the client the threshold for having to act to reduce risk is lower. She didn't presently report acting on her delusions. Although she had hit the other worker before losing her job, but in her current circumstances she didn't report feeling like acting on her experiences. Sometimes it is necessary to act to keep the client or others safe, but usually this will end the relationship as a place where psychological work can be done (as demonstrated in an earlier chapter). On the other hand, it's hard to be helpful to a client if one is in a state of anxiety about the possibility that the client might hurt herself or someone else).

She was reporting feeling less anxious about her experiences and that she had been dealing with conflict with her daughter more effectively. She now walked away if her daughter became aggressive towards her, rather than engaging with what she said, which had generally ended up in a fight.

After three months, we began delusion modification—that is a concerted attempt to evaluate the truth of her delusion. This was, it will be remembered, that she has discovered a secret, which had hitherto been kept from her, that there are secret meanings hidden in people's conversations and that she can communicate with people telepathically. I asked how she had come to know these things. She said that on reflection it had begun when she suspected her husband of having an affair while on holiday. She began to notice sexual innuendo in the things that he said to the woman she thought she was sleeping with. She might make a comment about something to eat and she would interpret it as really being a sexual invitation. Also, she remembered her late brother telling her that she (Tina) had a mental blockage about communication. This was when she first went to see a psychiatrist. This experience had clearly been present for many years, but she had begun to hear the double meanings more frequently recently. She came to believe that children learn this way of communicating from their parents. Every child had learnt this except her, and this is what her late brother was referring to, also she had the direct experience of hearing someone say something and hearing that it had two meanings. Hearing the double meanings wasn't really an interpretation, it was more like a changed experience. Just as hearing a voice is a changed experience not an interpretation. The other source of this belief seems to be that it explains the failures in her life. Now this isn't really evidence that the belief is true, and doesn't really fit with a straightforward cognitive account of her delusions, because it is a motivation rather than a reason to believe her delusion. One could suggest that the delusion improves her self-esteem. It is not that she is essentially unlovable, or that love doesn't exist, it is that she has lacked a particular skill. But I think that it was more that the delusion is a picture or expression of her deeply held belief that she is inferior. Behind this belief is, of course, a great sadness, disappointment, and despair.

The other source of evidence is her reinterpretation of things that have been said to her, for example, by her brother. Her brother had told her that she was going to "bring her up to date". She began to be sure that something was going on. She noticed her niece making comments about what was on TV or about the dog. She began to notice double meanings at work. The underlying message was that she was not acceptable or worthy, that she was lacking in understanding of other people. This underlying feeling about herself is, of course, understandable given what has happened in her life. She has early experiences of being ridiculed and belittled. Her family joined in with this and her parents are not able to protect her from the extended family. She has lost her husband, her older brother, and her job and she is alienated from her daughter. She may lose her house. The psychotic process involves concretisation. In place of feeling inferior, she perceives herself as lacking a particular skill. And her self-criticisms are externalised in that everyone else has the double meaning ability so she is the odd one out. This, of course, does not only occur in psychosis. In depression, Beck's negative cognitive filter involves (inter alia) seeing others as being negative towards oneself. But in Tina's case, this has become truly psychotic. Her self-criticism and doubt had been projected into other people and neutral comments are interpreted to fit with this and doubt is excluded. Actually, what makes this truly psychotic is the absolute lack of doubt, because there would be suspicious and near psychotic interpretations that would come near this. There is a dimensional element to this distinction. The perception of double meanings in what people say would be well explained by the cognitive model of delusions. If one is looking for this it is easy to find it, because of the inherent ambiguity of a lot of our language. As Tina projects more of her inner critical attacks into other people, she becomes surrounded by a hostile world. When she reacts to these perceived attacks, she generates an actual negative response from the world. She is sacked from her job for assaulting another worker; her husband divorces her when she accuses him of adultery saying that she needs help, and she doesn't have a partner. And these events can be further evidence of the reality of the attacks on her.

Some of these problems may be the result of her perception of others as rejecting or hostile. In Tina's case, the delusion seems to simply be a concretisation of her feeling that she is worthless. If Tina's delusions had been a dream, we would find it easy to link it to her life problems. One way to explain this is that Tina has undergone a regression in in relating to herself and the world. She experiences her fears and hopes as a perception of the external world, that is to say, her fears and self-criticisms have been projected out into the external world. They have been projected into other people. People are talking about her and making comments about her inferiority or are planning to harm her (her husband's affair). She believed that she was just seeing the truth about the nature of life. (I don't mean to imply of course that the nature of life is that the world is full of people who only had her best interests at heart!) She saw her family of origin as old fashioned and not in touch with the modern world and as not equipping her for life, which echoes her idea that she didn't understand an important aspect of communication.

She and I agreed that it would be useful to test out the truth of her beliefs. I suggested that her belief had certain negative consequences for her. It made her feel depressed that she had spent most of her life fundamentally not understanding what was going on and that it would be helpful to know if this was the case. I suggested the alternative hypothesis that her ideas were the result of her feeling depressed and that when people get depressed sometimes it affects their thinking. I normalised this by saying it was different to "going crazy". She knew that she had been depressed so this alternative hypothesis was acceptable to her.

We looked at alternative explanations for the evidence for her beliefs. I suggested that we test out her ability to communicate telepathically. I discussed confirmatory bias and selective attention and I suggested that she notice how often she heard references to "feathers" over the coming week, as a test of the power of selective attention, and to test out her powers of telepathy by trying to send out thoughts. At the next session, she had tried some of these ideas out. She had tried to test out whether she could really communicate telepathically by deliberately broadcasting her thoughts. She noticed that no one seemed to pick up on her thoughts. Furthermore, she had not experienced any incidents of double meanings in what people said. She had forgotten about the "feathers" experiment.

We discussed the result of her experiments in thought transference. She had found that trying to transmit thoughts didn't seem to have an effect. However, she thought that this was because these phenomena only worked when she was in a "receptive mood". This hypothesis, of course, makes perfect sense- why shouldn't a special psychic power depend on a particular state of mind? The logical problem here is, obviously, that without an independent measure of "receptivity" this hypothesis becomes un-falsifiable. However, this way of maintaining cherished hypotheses is arguably quite common in scientific thinking, and not just in delusional clients. It didn't seem productive to pursue this line of enquiry. Hazel Nelson (2005) suggests that it is important to have thought through and blocked these modifications in the belief prior to the crucial experiments being set up. Whether this would have made a difference, I don't know. She talked about always feeling that she lacked something, and how difficult it was to engage with a man if she couldn't converse due to her feeling of anxiety about having to read or write something down, and feeling that that at 52, she should be settled down with someone, not still looking for a partner. After this session it was the Christmas break. Her mood was still improved but her degree of belief in the double meanings and telepathy was still at 100%.

At the next session, I read her a text as a test of perceiving double meanings. I suggested that if we took a random text and she heard double meanings in the text this would imply that she could hear them when they weren't there. She agreed. I chose a text at random, and read a short passage. She heard double meanings in the text, but unfortunately concluded that these meanings were intended by the author. I showed her visual illusions to demonstrate that a perception can be faulty, and that what we see isn't always what is there. She found these illusions interesting, in particular the spiral illusion, but she didn't see that this made much difference to her belief.

The process of systematically evaluating her delusion had not progressed very far. Partly this was because when presented with evidence against her belief she responded by altering her belief to fit in with the evidence, thus protecting the delusion from falsification. And this is a quite normal way of protecting strongly held beliefs.

At the end of therapy, her mood had significantly improved. She was sometimes more able to be assertive with her son and her ex-husband. An important part of the therapy may have been the opportunity to talk through her problems with a sympathetic listener. She had no close confiding relationships, and she had no one to discuss her difficulties with. If she tried to talk about what she feared or believed she alienated others and got an invalidating response. Her delusional belief did not change. She developed a positive transference to me and this allowed me to work on her life problems in a more constructive manner.

One striking feature of her presentation is the parallel between her childhood trauma and her delusional belief. She had grown up believing that she was defective and the most obvious way that this was seen was in her inability to communicate by reading and writing. She now believed that she was ineffective in relationships because she had a defect in communication and had learnt how to decode the secret code others used and indeed, she had developed a special power of communicating without words. She did not see any parallel here. Her delusion expresses a deep, old personal wound but she is unaware of this.

As an example of delusion modification, Tina was not a success. However, in other ways her therapy was a success. Her problems with her delusion were an expression of her difficulties with relationships and her failures in her life. Here the psychodynamic conceptualisation is helpful as it put the delusional ideas in context, and this broadened my view of what the important goals in therapy with Tina might be. She had had the psychotic experiences for many years. As far as it is possible to tell they seem to have been triggered at a point in her life when she felt that her marriage was under threat. She had felt happy as a young mother and had found a way of overcoming her feelings of inferiority at work.

When she began to worry about her marriage, she became jealous and began to have psychotic experiences about hidden meanings. Her fears get confused with what she sees and hears. She knows she is fearful that her husband may be unfaithful to her and this is experienced both as a feeling and as a perception, and this is the psychotic transformation. It would have been useful to elaborate the circumstances surrounding the onset of this first episode. In any case, her old fears of being an outsider and defective were reignited, and the psychotic experience persisted. Developing a positive transference with the therapist was a counter to this central problem. Psychoanalysts might say that the negative transference has been avoided in the therapy, and that a better technique would have been to allow this to develop.

Reference

Nelson, H. (2005). *Cognitive therapy with delusions and hallucinations.* Cheltenham: Stanley Thornes.

14 Colin

Escape to a Marvellous World

Colin was a 50-year-old married man who had been referred to the City and Hackney psychological therapies department due to suicidal thoughts. Initially he was seen by a psychologist who focused on helping him with low mood. However, as he complained mainly of hearing voices, and as he didn't present with a consistently low mood he stopped seeing that psychologist and was referred back to the referral meeting for work with his psychotic symptoms. He had a diagnosis of schizoaffective disorder and a long history of difficulties in relationships.

He complained of hearing a voice which he believed to be a spirit, and which persecuted him by calling him insulting names and telling him that he was worthless, and saying other critical and threating things to him.

He lived with his wife and daughter. He had worked as a bookkeeper, which he had enjoyed, but he had not worked for several years. Previously, he had seen several other psychologists and had several different forms of psychological therapy. He complained of feeling depressed and of being harassed by the voice. Much of what the voice said to him was sexualised or pejorative. He believed in the spirit with 100% conviction. He had had a number of different diagnoses in the past and was on a range of different medications. He had developed the belief in the spirit some ten years previously. Over the years, he had learnt that talking about the spirit to his wife didn't get him anywhere, as she didn't believe it and got irritated by him talking about it. He was a regular member of a local socialist group at the community centre, where he had been going for years and he knew some of the people quite well. However, he had found that talking about the belief to other members of the group didn't get a sympathetic reception either so he had stopped mentioning it there.

Ten years earlier, he had gone to a meditation class and been taught several spiritual exercises using mantras and contemplating the void. It was in this context that he developed experiences of hearing voices. Although the class certainly promoted the idea of personal direct spiritual experience they had not suggested anything like his experiences to him. Was this an example of a socially acquired belief? And therefore, not delusional? As well as believing in spirits, he had the direct experience of hearing them.

DOI:10.4324/9781003168379-16

This didn't seem to be a belief that was acquired as part of cultural set of beliefs. It seems likely that the environment contributed to his beliefs in that he was encouraged to believe in unseen, spiritual realities and that ordinary, common-sense everyday reality is an illusion—that there is an unseen reality. Also, it is important here that this belief and these experiences persisted for years after he had stopped seeing anyone involved in the meditation class.

He had grown up in Romford as the youngest of a family of three children. He had a brother, who was 12 years older than him and a sister who was 10 years older than him. His brother had left the family by the time he was 10 and had emigrated to the USA. He recalled feeling that he was essentially an only child. He described his childhood as lonely. His father was from an upper middle-class background and his mother was working class. They had a difficult relationship and had few interests in common. His mother had had several brief affairs which further poisoned his parents' relationship. He found it difficult to relate to the other children at school and he was teased because of his stammer. He spent much of his time at school without any friends at all. He recalled having suicidal thoughts around the year after his brother had emigrated. He said that he had been sexually assaulted when he was a small child. He remembered this as part of the spiritual exercises. He, however, had no doubt about this. He felt alone, unacceptable, and unwanted. He didn't describe a close relationship with anyone as a child. He felt inferior and different to the other children at school. He felt on his own and without friends, and with a distant, unhappy family. The atmosphere at home was cold and undemonstrative, he said. His mother was unapproachable emotionally, so that when he had difficulties at school he was unable to go to her for help. He remembers thinking that all the other children were happy and it was just him that was out of step. He got the idea that he had not been wanted and had been an unwelcome surprise. He said that most of the children in the school were of Indian or Pakistani descent so that he was on the outside in not belonging to one of these groups. His stammer compounded his feelings of being an inferior outsider. He was quite good academically but he was teased and bullied about being studious. He began to get into fights at school as a way of dealing with his distress which only made the bullying worse. This resulted in the headmistress telling the children to leave him alone. Most of the time, he had no friends at all. No one around him was able to take effective action to help him with this problem, although the headmistress had tried. He spent most of his time alone in a fantasy world and no one noticed that he was unhappy, or if they did notice they didn't try and help him. He was admitted to hospital for the first time when he was 17 following an overdose.

As a young teenager, he had begun having casual sex with older men which in the short term made him feel wanted but ultimately made him feel lonelier. After leaving school he had gone to a technical college and had trained as a bookkeeper. He found work in a local firm and was happy doing this work. For the first time, there was something that he felt positive about in his life. He met his wife when he was in his mid-20s. When they met he had had one serious girlfriend who he had gone out with for a few months and she had not had any previous boyfriends. She wasn't very interested in sex, and they had more of a companionship. She was a committed socialist and feminist and she had persuaded him to become a socialist too, and this interest had continued up to the present.

After six or seven years he became dissatisfied in his marriage and had been feeling unhappy and depressed. At this time his daughter was five years old and he was now 33. He had seen a psychologist as a teenager when he began to self-harm. He hadn't found seeing the psychologist helpful, so he went to a meditation class. There were lectures on reincarnation, regression to past lives and on the role of negative karma in causing psychological problems and difficulties in relationships. The participants were encouraged to use meditation which would mostly help them to focus on the present and relax and also they were told that this would lead to a number of spiritual discoveries. During the classes, he discovered that he had committed sins in a past live which was why he had difficulties in his present life, and why he had had homosexual feelings. Bad things happened to him due to a spirit from another world wanting to get revenge on him. It was possible for him to talk to this spirit to release this negative karma. He met a young woman, Lorraine, at the classes who he discussed these experiences with. He began to believe that he and Lorraine would run off together. He said that the classes had had a positive effect on his life at this time, in that he self-harmed less, had less suicidal thoughts, and panicked less. (This is really a salutary story for psychotherapists. It is possible that any procedure which inspires hope, combined with a positive transference may have a beneficial effect on presenting symptoms.) However, although he became less angry, he also became less interested in his wife. This is obviously a negative result of the classes. His wife seemed to understand the process that was going on and she had a negative view of the meditation and his friendship with Lorraine. Colin became increasingly attached to her. He argued with his wife. Then he began to hear voices and see visions telling him to kill his wife and to kill himself. This was the first time that he had had these symptoms. So, the classes were now having a negative effect on his life. These discoveries rationalised his self-harm and sexuality, including his homosexual feelings. His sense of abandonment, he learnt, originated in having been given away by his parents in a previous life. Another negative effect was that he gave up work which gave him more time to focus on his spiritual experiences. It seems likely that here a set of psychotic experiences and beliefs are triggered by a spiritual exercise designed to encourage a belief in contact with spirits and an unseen realm. These experiences initially raise his self-esteem, by giving him a sense of importance and purpose, so they fulfil an unmet emotional need.

I will now present some transcripts from some of our sessions.

Therapy

First Session

He was very thin and wearing casual clothes. He gave the impression that he was eager to please. He began by explaining that he had seen several psychologists and counsellors previously. He went on to tell me that one counsellor (who he had seen through a Christian charity) had told him that she had to stop seeing him after a year as the service had adopted a policy of focusing on shorter term therapies. He went on to talk about how the counsellor had helped him with his depression by teaching him coping skills. He seemed more forlorn than angry about this ending. It seemed as though the end of therapy had been delegated to a policy decision so that he wasn't able to feel anything personal towards his counsellor about this ending. After all, it wasn't the counsellor that had decided to stop seeing him, but the faceless organisation.

This seemed fairly clearly to be a comment in relation to the transference, given that this was one of the first things that he said to me. I suggested that maybe he wondered about whether the counsellor had not really wanted to continue to see him. He agreed with this and went on to say that he was worried about being abandoned by people, and it had happened before. I suggested that this might be a worry about me today as he was beginning to see me and maybe I would also tell him one day that he couldn't see me anymore. He agreed with this, and said that everywhere he went it felt the same.

Commentary

Here the issue of his feelings about the transference in the very first session is very close to the surface, and it seemed most appropriate to discuss this with him. This would often not be the case. Another aspect of dynamic technique is useful here to focus on understanding and naming his feelings. I could have simply told him that I wouldn't suddenly announce that the therapy was over without talking this through with him which, although it would be true, and would address his fear about our relationship, would avoid discussing these important feelings. This fear of abandonment turned out to be a major theme in his problems. Clients often do begin therapy with a re-enactment of their central problem.

Therapy began with a long period of engagement. After his initial worries about abandonment, he quickly settled in to talking quite freely about his problems. It was as though we had been working together for some time and he felt safe in the room with me. I noticed this and felt it was likely to be an avoidance of his worries, as it was painful for him to think about being unsafe, so that he acted as if that problem didn't exist (that is, the problem of having to negotiate a relationship with me). I didn't talk about this with him. The beginning of a dependant fear of being left was present at the start. Although the content of his delusion was, on the face of it, very negative, causing him considerable distress, there were aspects of his delusion which were positive for him. One of his spiritual beliefs when he had become delusional was that he was a saint.

His current beliefs in the voice, then, were influenced by a particular sub-cultural experience. You may think that his experiences at the meditation classes were encouraging him to engage with his fantasies rather than with the real world and, hence, were encouraging a withdrawal from reality and the experience of a psychotic view on the world.

A Later Session

Colin told me that after the previous session, he had been struggling with feelings of self-harm. The spirits had told him that I would dump him. He had felt upset after talking about his adolescent sexual experiences. The most upsetting thing had been talking about Lorraine. He had fallen in love with her and had been going to leave his wife for her. He told me that meeting the spirits when meditating had been a wonderful experience. The spirits had told him that he was destined for greatness. He was destined to be an important leader and to be involved in a new world order. The spirit had also told him that he was going to run away with Lorriane and be together with her. He said that he had met with her and that she had agreed to this (but it was unclear if this was in reality or in the spirit world, imagined through spiritual exercises). However, the spirits had turned against him. He had begun to think that the spirits were not all they claimed to be. He had told Lorraine that they were following the wrong light. She had said that "That is bullshit". He then went on to say that although his previous counsellor had told him that she had been told to stop seeing him, he didn't believe her as he knew some people who had seen her for longer.

Commentary

The main theme of this session seems to be his fear of abandonment, which turns up in different guises. He is probably not intending to link the spirit telling him that I was going to leave him to his being left by previous counsellors, because (he felt) they didn't find him worthwhile. His experiences and revelations had made him feel special and his friendship with Lorraine made him feel cared for. After all, in previous lives he had been important people. It was difficult to be sure what had actually happened with Lorraine and what had happened in his fantasies. In a state of self-hypnosis, he was told by a spirit that he would leave his wife and be with Lorraine. It wasn't clear to what degree she shared these ideas. When he left the classes and was at home, he began to experience voices and visions when not practicing meditation or any other spiritual exercises.

It is interesting to note that initially he found being involved with the meditation class very rewarding. Other people accepted him and he began to believe grandiose things about himself. He was told that he had been important people in a previous life and was destined to be an influential leader. His experiences seem to have given him an explanation of some of his problems which was blame-reducing. He had done bad things not because of a moral fault but because of who he had been in a previous life. Bad things happened to him as part of a process of expunging sinful or hurtful action from the past. Furthermore, he felt accepted and valued as he had never felt before. The spirits were going to get rid of his wife so that he could be with Lorraine. However, after leaving the group and returning home he became progressively more depressed and had increasing thoughts of self-harming.

Other people including his family increasingly saw him as unwell. At the meditation group, they told him to start taking medication. He began to feel that the meditation exercises had put him in touch with demonic rather than positive spiritual forces and that he had largely been deceived. So, the experience ended as a re-enactment of his previous experiences in his family and at school, of being rejected and found unacceptable. He ended up in hospital. The belief that he was in touch with demonic forces persisted following his discharge.

Explaining his problems by externalising them places his recovery in someone or something else. This preserves hope about his life and his future by projecting hope into these ideas or people. His later belief of being in touch with demonic forces is in some ways the same, in that there are powerful beings outside of himself which are closely involved in his life, only now it is the bad inner persecutor which is projected out rather than his hopes and aspirations. Now there is a different externalising process. For example, he now thought that he had been promiscuous, or thinking of leaving his wife because he was under the influence of the Devil. When he left the meditation group, he saw that the exercises got him in touch with the work of the Devil and saw the spirits as the agents of the Devil. He projected not just dangerous impulses but also aspects of himself into these beings. He rid himself of punitive guilt by projecting it into an external being.

Does this conceptualisation help? In the past psychologists have taught him coping skills and worked on helping him to accept his situation using mindfulness, which had helped but had been nowhere near as transformative as his experiences in the meditation classes. The belief in the good spirits and his glorious future, if the conceptualisation is right, is an attempt to redeem himself from his problems. At the beginning of therapy with me, he is hoping to have this in the sessions with me. The previous psychological work had disappointed him—he felt that the previous counsellor had wanted to get rid of him but had not been straightforward about this. The pattern is of hoping for an idealised positive relationship only to be disappointed and find himself being rejected, abandoned and despised.

He felt that the idealised contact with the meditation class was dangerous but more rewarding than the contact he had had since then. It was important to think about this at the beginning of therapy. His fears about being not interesting enough for me seem understandable given this context.

A Later Session

He rated his belief in the reality of the spirits at 100%. He said that he had been feeling more depressed than usual. His mood had dropped at the weekend but he didn't know why. The spirits had been giving him a lot of trouble, by making negative comments to him. The spirits had been telling him that I wasn't interested in him and suggested that I might be more interested in sex. I replied that these feelings were very common in therapy. I suggested that feeling more depressed might relate to talking more about his feelings. I said that he feels that he is lost in a mid-life crisis and finds it hard to think of goals, because he doesn't know where he wants to go.

Commentary

The development of the transference here re-enacts his relationship outside of therapy. The sessions begin with his anxiety about being abandoned by his previous therapist. He also had concerns about how long I am going to be able to work with him for. By the time that he is several months into the therapy, his voices are telling him that I am uninterested in him and that the solution is to seduce me to get my attention. This pattern of relationships is evident in his personal history. This idea is projected out into the spirits. As Malan (1995) points out there are degrees of unconsciousness about motives. At one end of the spectrum here he might consciously put into the mouth of the spirit something that he doesn't want to admit to. Alternatively, the idea could be just below the surface or so deeply hidden that he would feel perplexed and confused at the idea that it might relate to him. How to respond to this depends partly on how the client feels about these feelings or motives and that is closely linked to what degree they are unconscious. When I suggested that these feelings are common in therapy, he saw what I meant rather that rejecting this. If I had not felt that he would be likely to see this I would not have made the link. I said that feelings of insecurity were a normal part of therapy. Often with psychotic symptoms this type of suggestion does seem to the client to be a non sequitur. His delusional system is an outcome of his unmet emotional needs. As a child he felt unloved and excluded and alone. As a teenager he becomes rebellious, sometimes acts to portray himself as foolish, identifying with the aggressor and controlling the bullying by enacting it, he becomes promiscuous in a self–defeating effort to feel wanted. Getting into fights as a child not just expresses his anger but also draws more opprobrium from others.

Obviously, there is an information processing component to the formation of the delusion. He concludes that there is a spirit because he hears a disembodied voice and believes that it is trying to harm him. There has also been a social effect on his beliefs in that he has been encouraged to treat fantasy as reality and to believe that he can contact spiritual realms. This also fits with an information processing model of his delusion; in this case the information is the opinions of others and the pressure to social conformity, which is really where most people's beliefs come from rather than direct experience. But in this case, the main factor in producing the belief seems to be that the voice is an expression of his belief rather than the other way around. This is an example of the presentation of thoughts as perceptions, part of the change in thinking, the concretisation of thought, in psychosis.

This does not mean that this belief could not be a target for delusion modification, of course, but if a delusion met an affective need, or if it expressed or symbolised some important conflict, it might be harder to modify. In this, delusions do not all have to be the same and, in terms of responding to cognitive challenging for example, it is clear that they are not all the same. "Delusion" may not be a natural kind and may be more akin to "sore throat" rather than "influenza", and the causes and maintaining factors may be different in different people.

Cognitively challenging whether the delusion was true could be a useful indication of the direction of causation here. However, Colin's delusion does seem motivated by emotional factors. He presents his involvement with Lorraine as idealised. He will be able to dump his wife and fly off to America with the ideal partner. The function of Colin's delusion seems to have changed. At the beginning, it is an ego-enhancing, wish fulfilment delusion. He will have a perfect relationship and his destiny is to be a hero fulfilling the hope of past lives when he was also a hero. The delusion functioned to maintain hope by being in a world in which he is accepted and loved and had a purpose. Later he came to believe that the things that he had been told were lies and that he had been deceived. Currently he thought that he was attacked by voices, however the purpose of the attack was to improve him personally and that was why God allowed this torment to go on, so although it was distressing to him to be tormented by the spirits, it was also a belief that had some benefits for him. In particular, he currently thought that the grandiose ideas that he had had were based on lies the spirits had told him.

It would have been possible here to attempt a partial modification of the delusion, so that the parts of the belief that caused his distress would be changed. The punishment that he believed the spirits inflicted on him was, he thought, ultimately a sign that God was active in his life on a day-to-day basis, so the positive aspect of this ego-enhancing belief need to be addressed.

A Later Session

He said that he had been seeing shadowy figures. He had seen them walking past the door of the bedroom. These were Shadow Men. Someone had walked past his room and he thought it was his wife, but then realised that it was some sort of spirit. I didn't say much to this apart from acknowledging that this must have been disturbing. I felt that it would have been have been unhelpful to get too excited about this, given his previous experience. (I mean the experience of the classes, encouraging him to lose touch with reality and which had validated that his psychotic experiences were of real spirits.) Usually, evaluating the person's delusional beliefs is central to cognitive therapy, in Colin's case he had a history of having a connection with people who encouraged his beliefs about spirits; it felt important to avoid this particular way of relating to him (not finding the idea of the paranormal version of his life more interesting than the sane, mundane but real version of his life). He then went on to say that he had been feeling depressed for a while. He had been avoiding the socialist group and other social situations. He was feeling burdened. And he had argued with his wife about the housework. He couldn't say why he was feeling like this.

Here there are two possibilities. One could address the delusion by preparing the client to evaluate the truth of the belief, by listing the advantages and disadvantages of the belief being true, or by working on building up coping skills to deal with his visual, auditory, and somatic hallucinations. But in this case, this didn't seem a good idea given the conceptualisation and given his history of engaging with the delusion. It seemed likely that that focusing on the delusions and hallucinations might be counter-productive. There were clear elements of positive consequences in holding the delusion and with Lorraine an intense erotic transference had built up around exploring these experiences. Furthermore, he did have other problems which were more reality based, for example, his wife didn't do any of the housework and he had given up his job which had been a source of satisfaction to him. He had difficulties relating to other people at the socialist group. So, it made more sense to start working with him on these issues, as Colin had real-world problems to work on and as he wasn't totally lost in his delusional world.

I asked him more about when the low mood had begun. It had begun a few weeks ago. He had had trouble getting motivated. He then went on to say that he used to work as a bookkeeper but that nothing seems to work out in life. He had wanted to do something on the stage or in movies, but when he didn't get into stage design, he had trained in bookkeeping instead. He then went back to talking about the spirits who had said that they had ripped out his soul. He didn't draw any analogy here so I pointed out that the spirits wanting to rip out his soul reminded me of how he had felt about all the enterprises in his life, including his marriage. He listened to this and said that that was right. Indirectly of course this kind of comment can constitute a challenge to the truth of the delusional belief. In this example, it is difficult not to see the voices comments and his feelings of defeat as related. Furthermore, that he brings up the spirits when he is talking about the feelings of defeat suggests an unconscious association of themes. This phenomenon is important to listen out for because the client is communicating more than he knows. That is, unconsciously he links the two feelings or situations but consciously he is unaware of the link. Why, one might ask does he not see this link? This suggests an active avoidance of these feelings or the link between the feelings.

A Later Session

It had been a good week. His problem is his wife. Things are difficult with her and he had thought about the time when he had been going to go off with Lorraine to the USA. This line of thinking had been stopped by the spirits who injected painful things into his body and he smelt the smell of death. He had felt possessed.

Here his problem is his flesh and blood relationship with his wife. But there is the memory of the possibility of the relationship with Lorraine which was only prevented by the intervention of evil. The delusion functions as an explanation for the failure of his relationship with Lorraine. This is an example of splitting. Lorraine is good and he would have been good with her. A bad force had intervened to prevent him from being good. This however, has a defensive function. He can preserve the fantasised good relationship with Lorraine because it is unattainable. The hope of good is preserved by being projected out, while he is left with his real and despised and despising wife. The other theme here as he is explaining this situation to a therapist is, of course, how it relates to the transference. As in a previous session the spirits had told him he needed to seduce me in order to keep me interested the fear of abandonment had been present in our sessions from the beginning.

I thought that describing this to him would not be helpful so I said something about his feeling that he didn't get his needs met and that he felt like there was a force that always stopped him from getting what he wanted, which was near enough a paraphrase of what he had said to me, although omitting the demonic part of the description.

Over the next eight sessions I continued to engage him with active listening. Two stories emerged. In his present circumstances, he had a difficult relationship with his wife. She was often not interested in sleeping with him. This made him feel unloved. At the same time, he talked about his aging father's health, his admissions to hospital and his frustration that his sister left this up to him. It sounded like because he lived nearer, the responsibility for checking on his father and visiting him when he was unwell defaulted to him. At the same time, he was also accosted by spirits who told him that he was bad or worthless and unloved. As well as this account of his current situation he also told me about the circumstances surrounding the development of his delusion.

In any event, what he brought as problems in the sessions were primarily his difficulties with his life-the two strands in the conversation were explaining his story and telling me about his day-to-day difficulties. These alternated and it seemed important in his case to be more interested in reality than in insanity.

Reference

Malan, D. (1995). *Individual Psychotherapy and the science of psychodynamics*. London: Butterworth Heinemann.

15 Amara

Hidden Suspicions—All Occasions Do Inform Against Me

Amara was referred to the psychological therapies department at Stone House Hospital in Kent. She was a woman in her late 30s and was referred for work on her chronic delusion that she was being conspired against. She had been seen by the mental health team since her first breakdown when she was in her early 20s. She had a diagnosis of schizophrenia. She was brought up in Ethiopia and lived there until her family emigrated to the UK when she was 10 years old. Her father had been involved in some criminal activity, and with a militia, and they had emigrated to the UK mainly due to his past. She remembered her father as a violent man who used to hit her and her mother. When I met her, she worked regularly in a sheltered workplace and had a number of friends whom she saw quite regularly, most of whom she had met through the mental health service. She lived alone in a rented flat.

I saw her initially for a number of assessment sessions. She had memories of her parents arguing and they had broken up when she was 16. Her father had always been involved in illegal activity and she remembered when she was a small child the house being raided by the police, looking for her father and feeling confused and scared. Her father was also involved with a militia and would sometimes go away for several weeks. Her earliest memories were of conflict between her parents. She remembered being sent by her mother to collect her father from a café or bar. Eventually her father moved out to live with his girlfriend. As therapy progressed her description of her father became darker. Her mother remarried after a year or two. She got on well with her stepfather. Her two brothers were considerably older than her. She remembered feeling alone in that she was the only daughter and also the baby of the family.

At school, she had enjoyed art, PE, and woodwork. There were no other children from her background at the school and this made it hard to fit in. In year 11, she came to think that people at school were talking about her. This got her into fights and she was eventually expelled. After she was expelled, she took an apprenticeship. She had her first breakdown at 18, and she had been admitted to hospital. When she was acutely ill, she would think that she was getting messages from the TV and that other people's gestures had hidden threatening meanings.

DOI:10.4324/9781003168379-17

She summarised her delusional belief as "People want to hurt me"; "People are plotting to kill me"; and "People have a bad intention towards me". The evidence for her suspicions was an intuition, or that she picked up a "vibe". Amara's delusions involved a projection of an inner persecutory object into other people and also into chance events. She was able to work and she had a circle of friends so she was engaged with other people—but the depth of her relationships with her friends was often superficial and she had difficulties sustaining a relationship. She saw her friends when they came around to drink and she often harboured suspicions about them of one sort or another. As well as being suspicious about people she also would think that in some way events worked against her or persecuted her. For example, she thought that if she watched her football club play that this would make them lose. This didn't seem to be through somebody making this happen but more like fate was conspiring against her. (Later in the therapy she began to believe that there was a particular family that was involved in making things go wrong for her, but when I first saw her, she hadn't settled on a particular group.)

She also complained of having difficulties sustaining a relationship with a man, and this was a major problem for her. After I had known her for nearly a year, she confided in me that had initially thought that when I went to see her, I was coming to spy on her. I asked her why, in that case, she had agreed to see me and she said that it was so she could keep an eye on me. At the beginning of therapy, I had no idea about this.

One source of "evidence" for her belief was that when things went badly for her, she tended to ascribe it to the malevolent motives of some group, and when she thought back she remembered these interpretations as facts. So, if her football team lost when she watched them she would explain this as due to the universe frustrating her and then later, when she looked back she would remember it as an example of the universe frustrating her and evidence that this was the case.

At one point she was injured in a car accident and seriously hurt. Immediately after this event she explained it in a reality-based way- the other driver had gone through a red light by being distracted. After some time, however, she began to think that it had been planned as part of a conspiracy and that she had been set up. It was as if immediately after the event she was clear about the detail of the attack and this provided sufficient explanation, as the detail faded it was easier to fit the event into her paranoid beliefs. And this served to maintain her belief.

Engagement

First Session

I saw her at her home. She welcomed me and offered me coffee. She was friendly and talkative. I explained who I was and why I was there and asked her to tell me how she was. She said "People are against me". She went on to say that her friends weren't against her but other people were. At that time, I didn't take this as a possible reference to me, although looking back on it I'm not really sure why I didn't. She told me that people play games. She thought that people wanted to kill her. This, unsurprisingly, made her very anxious. I asked her about her childhood and she said that she had two brothers who were much older than her. Her parents were always arguing and she remembered her father getting furiously angry and smashing things up, and hitting her mother. It had been really frightening for her. When she left school she had an apprenticeship, but then she got put on medication and she slept all day, and had to give it up. Following this she had had six admissions to hospital.

I asked her how she knew that people were wanting to harm her. She said one thing was that when she goes out people don't want to talk to her. She said this campaign against her had got so bad that she has tried to kill herself a few times. She said that she works most days but she no longer goes out much in the evening, but stays home. I suggested that it would be good to meet with her for a while to get to know her before thinking about how I might help her, and arranged to return the following week.

Second Session

She invited me in and offered me coffee. We sat in her living room and she began to talk without further ado. She had gone out to a bar in the week. A man had bumped into her. She thought he had probably done it deliberately and that this was part of the general campaign of hatred against her. She hadn't reacted but it was an example of how people hated her. Also, when she is driving with her boss, he doesn't talk to her and she thinks this shows that he is against her. When she talked to her friends about her boss's behaviour they told her that that was how the boss was with everyone, and it wasn't just her. They said that often people aren't overtly friendly at work but it doesn't mean that they are hostile to you. She obviously didn't really believe this as she went on to say that if she were a drug dealer or a criminal, she would understand the persistent animosity. She went on to talk a little about her family. Her brothers were 10 and 11 years older than her, so she had never really felt close to them growing up. She had always been the baby sister. She told me that she was close to her stepfather and that her biological father had died four years previously. Her stepfather was a good man.

She said that the beginning of all the trouble was when she was at school and her closest friend had begun to talk about her behind her back. She felt that people were jealous of her which was why they had talked about her at school. And she felt it was still the same; people talked about her, or were hostile to her out of envy.

Commentary

In this session, Amara gave some examples of current evidence for her belief. She seems to interpret anything that isn't overt friendliness as hostility and, furthermore hostility with intent to kill her. This seems to be an example of confirmation bias. Because she believes that people seek to harm or kill her she sees hostility in every action that isn't overtly friendly. She said a little about what had been going on in her life when the delusion developed. In her case, she was trying to fit in to a different culture, with little support at home as her parents were at war with each other and she felt like an only child, being the only girl and the baby of the family. There is the beginning of frank paranoia in the feeling that others are talking behind her back at school.

When she mentions the two father figures in her life there is a split between good and bad. Why does she mention this in this session? This is her second session with her therapist and this can be taken as an unconscious communication about her feelings about her therapist. Is the therapist going to be her father or her stepfather? It seems likely that she is wondering about this early on in her therapy. After all, she told me that, apart from her friends, people want to harm her. It didn't feel at the time that she was anxious or suspicious about me, but as it later transpired, she *was* feeling suspicious about me and that fits with the hypothesis that the talk about her stepfather and father is a reference to who I will turn out to be. At the time I was unaware of this aspect of our relationship. This would have been useful to think about, not to interpret this to her, but being aware that under her friendly exterior there were indeed highly suspicious feelings would have influenced how I approached her.

The Third Session

At the next session, she said that she had been to the club and that everyone had been friendly. She had seen some of her friends there. She went on to tell me that all her friends had mental illnesses. I asked how she knew that if people didn't talk to her, they were feeling hostile towards her and she said it was based on "vibes". She went on to say that sometimes she feels unwanted by her family. Her mother and brothers lived a short distance away but she didn't see them that often, and she felt that her having a mental illness had affected how they see her. She said that her father had been aggressive and had beaten her and that if she cried her father would beat her harder. Her mother used to send her out to get her father when her father was drunk. Her father had been involved in serious crime which is why they had had to emigrate.

Commentary

Her feeling of being in danger may relate to her early childhood trauma. She felt unsafe as a small child. She had been beaten by her father and had seen her house raided by the police looking for her father. She had witnessed conflict between her mother and father. This doesn't mean that these experiences have caused her later paranoid belief, of course. The vast majority of people who experience domestic violence as children do not develop paranoid delusions, but it may be part of the cause, given other factors. Also, it's important to note that her understanding of people is very black or white and that this is very concrete for her. If people don't like her then they want to kill her. They hate her because they are envious of the good things that she has. On the other hand, she has chosen to share some of these painful experiences and feelings with me, which is a sign that she is beginning to develop some trust in me. In terms of the cognitive model, her beliefs are maintained by interpreting the evidence in the light of her beliefs and then taking it as evidence that the belief is true.

I am continuing to engage her by listening to her. This is not a neutral process. Most people she meets will tell her quite quickly that she is wrong about what she believes. What I have missed however (and would have been good not to have missed), is the unconscious message behind the friendly front. I continued to see her for a month listening to what had been happening in her life and putting together the beginnings of a conceptualisation.

Beginning of Therapy

Working on Her Depression

A month later she explained to me that when people cough it is a sign. One person is signalling to another about her, using the cough. Also, there are cameras in the house. She knows this because people repeat things that she has said, or make allusions to thinks she has said or thought. She doesn't understand how this works but she thinks that this shows that she is being monitored.

She repeated that people don't speak to her. If she goes to a club, men don't come up to her. She noticed that her friends don't get attention from men either. People always cough when she is around so she is sure that it is a negative comment on her. The other day her friend rubbed her jaw (the friend's own jaw that is) and Amara got a sore jaw. She found this mystifying because she hadn't worked out how the friends jaw had made her jaw ache. She went on to reflect that people had ignored her all her life. This isn't on the face of it linked to what she had been talking about. But of course, it is possible to link this. Both her feelings of suspicion and paranoia and her sense of never having been noticed by people are examples of feeling that she has never been wanted.

Commentary

Now here she speaks about bizarre delusions and experiences. These bizarre delusions and experiences shade into her general life and her more ordinary fears about other people. As she gets more comfortable with me she lets me know about stranger experiences—her experience that the boundaries of herself could be broken and the experience that she is as the centre of attention from everyone. I decided that it would be better to begin by working on her mood rather than her psychotic symptoms, because we both agreed that these were problems and she had problems in her life that we could address. Her delusion is obviously a source of distress to her, but probably better addressed when the rapport between us was stronger.

To work on her depression, I asked her to keep a diary of her mood; I asked her to note when her mood got worse, how bad it was on a 7-point scale, and what was going on at the time. I taught her progressive muscle relaxation and suggested that she try this out at home. I didn't at this stage share any conceptualisation with her because I doubted that she would accept it as a possibility and, worse, that she would think I wasn't taking her concerns and fears seriously.

The Next Session

In the next session, she told me that she hadn't kept a mood diary. She found that the relaxation exercises helped in the office but she hadn't done them at home. She said that she had been feeling anxious most of the time. She had been thinking about people wanting to harm her a lot. She had been to a nightclub and felt that everyone was looking at her. She said that she heard voices in the nightclub and then saw people listening to these voices that she was hearing, confirming that these were real voices rather than figments of her imagination. I continued to try to lift her mood mainly using behavioural techniques of activity scheduling and focusing on strengths rather than problems. But her delusional ideas were central to her reports of her experiences. She talked more freely about her paranoid ideas, which is again a deepening of trust in me.

Delusion Modification

Some three months later, I began working on modifying her delusions. I suggested that it might be worth checking out if she was correct because if the doctors account was correct, she was having a lot of distress that she didn't need and having her life restricted unnecessarily. She believed the doctors when they told her she had schizophrenia so setting up the hypothesis that she might be mistaken in her belief that she was being conspired against was relatively easy. I asked her to note examples of when people slighted her. As an alternative explanation I suggested that her parents' hostile marriage and her father's aggression and physical abuse of her, her father's involvement with a militia, the general background of political violence and then later emigration and the bullying friend at school could have led to the belief that other people could be dangerous and that she could be vulnerable, and this could have led to her up to be suspicious of other people.

The Next Session

She hadn't recorded examples. She told me that a man at the working men's club liked her. She went on to say that she thinks that she doesn't have a boyfriend because "people have it in for me". She couldn't think of any evidence relating to this. A man at the club had asked her why she didn't have a boyfriend. She has the feeling that there are cameras and bugs in her house. I put the alternative explanation that she didn't have a boyfriend as she avoids talking to men. I also asked her how her theory fitted with the man asking why she didn't have a boyfriend? She listened to these alternative explanations without rebutting them but without taking them up.

A Later Session

Some weeks later she told me that she may have a boyfriend. A man at the club asked her to come around for tea. She feels that people know who is and talk about her. She thinks that her life gets shown on TV. She thinks that there is a screen which is about where she has been seen. When she was walking down the street people were looking at her. They cough—but it isn't a proper cough. She feels that they look down on her. We went through alternative explanations of these experiences,

Commentary

Modifying the delusion was having little impact on her; however, she is engaged in the therapy and has started to engage more with life. Although I had been suggesting that she should try to take on activities to lift her mood, I hadn't suggested that she should go out to the club more often. I had suggested that she might be without a partner because she avoided men and now she seemed to be talking to men. As she engages in therapy she is engaging more in her life. Also, she is telling me more detail about her psychotic experiences as she begins to trust me more.

Following this session, she was involved in a car accident and was injured badly enough that she ended up in hospital. At first this was, she thought just bad luck. But after a couple of weeks, she started to think that the crash had been planned.

A Later Session

She told me that she had gone on a date but it had gone badly. All her friends had joined her and the man had run off. She hadn't invited her friends so she said it felt like bad luck. I had suggested that she should try to tape the coughing when she went out. She had gone to the shops with the intention of taping the coughing but there hadn't been any. Over the next few sessions, as I asked her to collect evidence about the coughing, she said that she hadn't noticed it. It doesn't seem likely that this was an effect of therapy. Trying to keep notes on the coughing is not likely to have reduced the number of people who were coughing around her. In a later session, the man who had not come on the date had got angry with her. I continued to suggest that she record evidence she has for her belief.

Commentary

In these sessions, I rather single-mindedly persist with asking her to record evidence for evidence for her delusional belief. I focus on coughing as it is the most tangible of the evidence that she presents, looking back on these sessions I think I should probably have changed tack earlier. I was focused on the delusion as this seemed to permeate all of her experiences in a way that poisoned them. However, she was also going out and trying to engage with other people which she had not been doing previously, and this seems a really important improvement.

A Later Session

However, in the next session, she had begun to observe the examples of the coughs she heard, so maybe the persistence was worthwhile. She noticed a chef coughed once but was otherwise friendly, and she realised that this was a counter-example to her theory about coughing being a form of signalling. She went on to say that she was generally treated badly by people. They laugh at her. They have picked on her. At school, no one would talk to her. She was still not working due to the injuries from her accident and she said that she has less money now as she is not working so she is unable to go out as often. She had noticed that women stare at her in the street, and that they were watching her with hostility. This was when she told me that it had been hard to trust me at the beginning.

Commentary

In this therapy, the attempts at modifying her delusion appear to have started to introduce some doubt in that she noticed that the chef whose coughing had aroused her suspicions seemed in other ways friendly, which runs counter to her paranoid idea that the coughing indicates a malicious communication about her. Of course, she could have chosen to stick to her belief in the maliciousness of the communication and interpreted the friendliness as subterfuge, so that she didn't is not determined by her noticing this fact. Rather it seems that she can notice this inconsistent fact because it seems possible to her. A notable feature is that as the sessions progress Amara is able to confide increasingly in the therapist. She talks about progressively more paranoid experiences and interpretations and by the end of this series of sessions she is able to let me know that she didn't trust me at the beginning of the therapy. Ironically this demonstrates an increasing degree of trust. Her main schemas relate to mistrust and abuse, so this is a contrasting experience, which is of therapeutic gain.

16 Sheila

The Wronged Wife—Repetition of Loss

Sheila was referred to the Psychological Therapies department in Hackney for cognitive therapy for psychosis. She had a chronic, medication resistant, delusional belief that her ex-husband had swindled her out of money and had been having an affair with another woman. She had been medically retired from the Civil Service after having been depressed for two years. Her depression had been moderately severe and had led to her being unable to work effectively, so eventually she was discharged on a full pension. However, although her mood improved after she left the civil service, and she had no financial worries, she remained depressed. She found it impossible to adjust to not working.

She had not had any psychiatric symptoms before this breakdown. She got depressed during a difficult conflict at work. She had been working in IT and a new manager was appointed who was critical and demanding. This evolved into frank bullying, where her boss told her to hide things from other staff members and took credit for her work as well as being relentlessly critical. She had complained about her boss but this had inflamed the situation. In the middle of this conflict, her mental health declined. Although her husband had been supportive during the conflict at work, once she left work their relationship quickly declined and they separated and divorced after a year. She had been married for ten years prior to this. Soon after this, she had become involved with another man and moved away from Manchester to London.

Later she interpreted what had happened around her marriage breakdown in a different way. She ended up believing that her ex-husband had lied to her and deceived her about a number of important things. She came to believe that he had inherited a fortune from a distant relative, that he had been having an affair with another woman while they were still married. He hadn't told her about the inheritance so that she wouldn't make a claim on the money. It really hurt her to realise that he had been unfaithful to her, and had moved in with the other woman as soon as she was out of the picture. She had no real evidence to support this belief and, although there is nothing bizarre about these ideas, the way she supported these ideas marked them out as psychotic.

She had two younger brothers. Her parents had lived in the country in Yorkshire. She remembered her parent's marriage as very conservative. Her

DOI:10.4324/9781003168379-18

mother had not gone out to work. Her parents' expectations of her were that she would marry and have children and, as she was a woman, they didn't think that her having a career was important. When she was 10 years old, her father had been made redundant and had been around at home with her for about a year before he got a job in the South. Her had moved away but her had her mother had stayed behind and eventually they divorced. She hardly ever saw him after he moved. During this time her father had been at home, and she had become close to him. She had responded to this loss by behaving badly for a period of time. No one seemed to talk to her about what had happened. After her parent's divorce her mother found work and externally things settled down quickly. There were no financial difficulties. When she was 12 her mother remarried and her step-father moved into the house. Her relationship with her step father was fine at the beginning but deteriorated as she grew into a young woman. As a teenager she had been an outsider. She hadn't fitted in with the others at school and felt second best to her brother at home. She had become active in the local church group at 14. She had found this gave her somewhere where she fitted in.

Without much encouragement from her family, she had done well at school, gone to university, entered the Civil Service as a fast-tracked graduate and had done extremely well professionally. She said that she had been motivated to do well as a retaliation against her mother and step-father's lack of ambition for her.

She and her ex-husband moved in together when she was 25. They moved away because she wanted to get away from family and the friends she had at the time, after 5 years together they got married. She devoted a lot of her energy and time to her career. They had had plans to have a child but it was never the right time, due to work commitments. When the problems started at work everything began to implode. She went off on long-term sick leave, her husband was doing things on his own and they began to be more distant with each other. They agreed to separate.

When they separated, she moved away to the south of England. After six months she contacted her husband and wanted to talk to him to resolve her feelings. He wasn't interested in talking to her. She turned up at his house and in the ensuing argument she threatened him. After that, they had no contact with each other at all. After about eight months she met her new partner and began a relationship with him. One day, she bumped into an old friend who told her that her ex-husband had moved in with someone else and had come into a large inheritance. However, her ex-husband denied this and there was no other evidence that it was true. She became depressed, her ex-husband was unwilling to meet with her after the scene she had caused previously and, feeling everything was hopeless, she tried to end her life. When she was depressed her delusion about her husband's inheritance, and her husband having been unfaithful preoccupied her and she felt sad about this most of the time. She believed that her ex-husband had tried to tell her about the affair when they were together by hinting. She had worked this out by going over their remembered conversations. Also, she said that her friends had told her about these things, but that now they denied that they had said these things to her. She thought that there had been legal action taken to ban people from talking about it. She had wondered what to do about it and had considered legal action but in the end had decided not to do this.

Although her mood was much improved from the time she first came in contact with the mental health service, she was still depressed, so we agreed to work on her mood using CBT. She said that she lacked motivation to do anything. She saw her current partner irregularly as he lived in Scotland. She had no work and although she had a comfortable pension she felt at a loss without work. I began by giving her an activity schedule to complete. She filled this in and increased her activity levels. A number of negative events occurred which contributed to her mood remaining low. A letter she had written to her ex-husband was returned "not known at this address". She said that being out of work was particularly difficult as she generally had high standards for herself, and thrived on achievement. In the past, this had worked for her, but now it wasn't working and she felt "brought down like human garbage". The psychiatrists talked to her about her diagnosis being delusional disorder or schizophrenia. Unfortunately, this was not acceptable to her. Having perfectionistic standards and having been successful in work and in her social life did not sit easily with having been medically retired let alone with a psychotic diagnosis. She could not accept the possibility that she could have been so radically out of touch with reality, and the anxiety of this possibility increases her motivation to maintain the truth of the belief.

Hazel Nelson (2005) describes delusions as being maintained by anxieties about the implications of the belief being false. (1) The anxiety about having a mental illness, (2) the anxiety about having been out of touch with reality, and (3) the anxiety of having been psychotic. These possibilities threaten (1) self-esteem, (2) the person's confidence in their own judgement, and (3) a secure future. This is a version of the idea that a symptom is maintained as a defence. In Sheila's case, whatever the origins of the delusion, it was certainly maintained by a fear of the personal implications of it being true. This generated a negative relationship with her psychiatrists, who tried to explain the illness that she had had to her. Although the idea of self-deception is, of course, a commonplace, and hardly restricted to those with mental health problems, it is evidence for the unconscious, or for splitting of the self that it is possible to be motivated to not believe something because of the consequences of believing it.

A Session

Over the next few weeks, she began to use distraction to deal with her mood. She read books, watched videos, went walking, talked to her partner on the phone and played with the cat.

As her mood improved, she began to worry about her current relationship. Her partner was working in Scotland and it was difficult to see how they could live together. She woke in a cold sweat gripped by the fear of not finding work. She had not found work mainly, she thought, because she now had a history of having being admitted to a psychiatric hospital. This was progress. Rather than being preoccupied by her delusion about her ex-husband she was now preoccupied and anxious about a reality-based problem. Her therapy proceeded along the lines of a cognitive therapy of a depressed client who was not psychotic. At times she did struggle with suicidal thoughts and feelings. When she didn't find it easy to find work, she arranged to do some work with a friend of the family which provided her with a reference.

I began working with her on her depressed thoughts and interpretations of events using straightforward cognitive challenging. This helped. For example, she thought at one time "I am in a hole and I can't get out". We looked at this in relation to her past achievements I asked if it was true that she couldn't get out of the hole that she was in and, as she said that in the past she had overcome a number of different difficulties. This lifted her mood. She was able to use this technique at home using a thought record and this did improve her mood. In my experience, this is quite unusual in clients with chronic delusions. Her suicidal feelings were exacerbated when she blamed herself for mistakes she had made. She blamed herself for having been unfaithful to her ex-husband and this guilt could develop until she felt that she didn't deserve to live. However, her mood gradually lifted.

A Later Session

Some weeks later, she began the session by saying that her boyfriend wanted more commitment and is asking why she can't get past the issues about her ex-husband. Her ex-husband rang her and said that it wasn't true that he had come into an inheritance or had an affair. She didn't believe him, but wanted to be able to move on and leave her feelings behind.

A Later Session

She continued to rate her degree of belief in the inheritance as "100%". She got depressed about what had been happening and had spoken to a friend of a friend who knew a man who claimed to be her ex-husband, although he didn't look like her ex-husband, and had recently become a father.

A Later Session

Her mood lifted. She sent a letter to her ex-husband at his mother's address. He had rung her feeling outraged and said that it was all untrue. He contacted her parents. Her parents had believed him. However, she was sure that he was lying. She found herself thinking about her delusional beliefs almost all the time. She said she wanted to move on from it all. She felt hurt that her parents believed her ex-husband rather than her. She ruminated about ways to get justice. Here her delusional belief pushes other people further away from her. And by pushing people away she avoids alternative perspectives on what happened. The story about the man who said that he was her ex-husband but didn't look like her ex-husband sounds if there is some misunderstanding or confusion. The possibilities that come to mind are that the person giving this information had misidentified Sheila, and is talking about someone else, or that Shelia's friend has misunderstood the information. Emotionally her delusion cuts her off from those around her which makes it easier to come up with the hypothesis she was being deceived. This would have alienated her further from her parents, which in turn would have left her with less information about the reality-based world, and more isolated and more alone.

Delusion Modification

She said she would like to be free of all of this so I considered delusion modification with her. This was after spending two months of cognitive therapy to lift her mood. Although the cognitive strategies of challenging negative thoughts and assumptions worked for her, a problem was that one of the sources of depression was the underlying delusional belief. So, it made sense to attempt to try to alter the delusion. It was of note that as her mood improved her conviction in, and preoccupation with the delusion did not decrease. It was, of course, important to have an established relationship with Sheila before suggesting examining the truth of the belief. I suggested to her that we could look at her beliefs about the inheritance or her ex-husband becoming a father to explore whether she was correct or not about these things. I pointed out that the belief caused her significant distress, and if it were not true there would be no need for the distress. But she clearly didn't think this was likely to be helpful and so I didn't pursue this line of therapy. I got the feeling that she felt that the possibility of her having been wrong about these things was a severe blow to her self-esteem.

Because of my intuition that it was going to be counter-therapeutic to push to explore whether the delusion was true or not, I turned to discussing the pros and cons of continuing the pursuit of the truth of the belief and not with the looking at the truth of the belief itself. While not exactly being a partial modification this is something akin to it.

We did a pros and cons analysis of continuing to try to get evidence for her belief. These pros and cons are all suggestions that she made. I didn't give her these ideas.

Advantages of Continuing to Try to Prove the Inheritance Existed

- she might be able to resolve the issue
- if she solved it, she would be rich
- she wouldn't need a job
- she will be able to travel to see her partner
- she wouldn't be thinking about it all of the time
- she would feel that she got justice

Disadvantages of Continuing to Try to Prove That the Inheritance Existed

- she's not moving forward in her life
- she's stuck in limbo
- her existence revolves around these two issues.
- she could spend years fruitlessly pursuing her goal

Advantages of Giving Up the Pursuit

she wouldn't feel like she was banging her head on a brick wall
she wouldn't get angry or depressed
she would have time and energy for other things
she wouldn't resent her parents not believing her

Disadvantages of Giving Up the Pursuit

loss of the inheritance
feeling that she failed
feeling that she wasted her efforts

I always find the degree to which clients can be aware of these advantages and disadvantages of their symptoms or patterns of behaviour slightly surprising. On reviewing these points, she felt that she would be better off giving up her attempt to prove the existence of the inheritance. But this, of course, was easier said than done.

In the end, the therapy stopped when Shelia fell out with her psychiatrist and asked to be discharged. She wanted to continue to see me but I explained that this would not be possible outside of the multidisciplinary team. Obviously here is an example of splitting, in that I am the good object and the rest of the team are the bad object. But the reality was that there wasn't an option for her to be seen. It would have been good if we had been able to find a private psychologist for her to see, but this was precluded by her lack of income.

There was a striking parallel between her delusional belief and the loss of her father at the age of 10. She had been particularly close to him for a year as he had been at home and not working. Then suddenly he had left and never came back. When she separated from her husband this was initially mutual but she ended up believing that he had betrayed and defrauded her. She isn't aware of any link here, and it is as if the delusion acts like an unsignalled memory. I become idealised in the transference and the mental health team are denigrated as part of the same process of splitting

Reference

Nelson, H. (2005). *Cognitive therapy with delusions and hallucinations*. Cheltenham: Stanley Thornes.

Index